中国慢性病预防控制能力调查报告

中国慢性病预防控制能力调查报告
2011

主　编　梁晓峰　施小明

副主编　翟　屹　司　向

编　者（按姓氏拼音顺序）

方益荣　绍兴市疾病预防控制中心
房玥晖　中国疾病预防控制中心营养与健康所
丁贤彬　重庆市疾病预防控制中心
梁晓峰　中国疾病预防控制中心
路　静　北京协和医学院公共卫生学院
施小明　中国疾病预防控制中心
司　向　中国疾病预防控制中心
唐雪峰　四川省疾病预防控制中心
翟　屹　中国疾病预防控制中心
朱晓磊　中国疾病预防控制中心
谢　晨　北京市疾病预防控制中心

中国协和医科大学出版社

图书在版编目（CIP）数据

中国慢性病预防控制能力调查报告. 2011 / 梁晓峰，施小明主编. —北京：中国协和医科大学出版社，2015.4

ISBN 978-7-5679-0309-8

Ⅰ. ①中… Ⅱ. ①梁… ②施… Ⅲ. ①慢性病-防治-调查报告-中国-2011 Ⅳ. ①R4

中国版本图书馆 CIP 数据核字（2015）第 071015 号

中国慢性病预防控制能力调查报告 2011

主　　编：梁晓峰　施小明
责任编辑：韩　鹏
助理编辑：杨小杰

出版发行：中国协和医科大学出版社
（北京东单三条九号　邮编 100730　电话 65260378）
网　　址：www. pumcp. com
经　　销：新华书店总店北京发行所
印　　刷：北京佳艺恒彩印刷有限公司

开　　本：787×1092　1/16 开
印　　张：10. 75
字　　数：200 千字
版　　次：2016 年 1 月第 1 版　　2016 年 1 月第 1 次印刷
印　　数：1—4000
定　　价：24. 00 元

ISBN 978-7-5679-0309-8

前　言

慢性非传染性疾病，简称慢性病，是一大类疾病的总称，主要指心脑血管疾病、癌症、慢性呼吸系统疾病、糖尿病等，其特点是病程长、流行广、致残致死率高、社会资源消耗多。随着我国疾病谱变化和人口老龄化的快速推进，以及工业化和城镇化进程的加快，我国慢性病发病人数在快速上升，调查时我国确诊的慢性病患者已超过 2.6 亿人，因慢性病导致的死亡占总死亡的 85%，导致的疾病经济负担已占总疾病经济负担的 70%，成为群众因病致贫返贫的重要原因。

慢性病预防控制能力可在一定程度上反映慢性病预防控制的应对情况，是慢性病预防控制工作发展的基础。中国疾病预防控制中心已于 2009 年和 2010 年开展了两次全国慢性病防控能力调查，并于第二次调查之前，开展了慢性病防控能力评估专题研究，系统梳理了国内外慢性病防控能力调查现状，建立了评估指标体系，形成了调查实施方案，定制了调查报告系统。前两次调查数据不仅为制定慢性病防控政策提供依据，也为深化医药卫生体制改革的评估工作提供参考依据。

本次调查仍然沿用 2010 年全国慢性病防控能力调查问卷，调查包括疾病预防控制机构和基层医疗卫生机构慢性病防控能力，同时还涉及卫生行政部门政策管理等内容，调查于 2012 年 9 月~2013 年 3 月进行，反映的是 2011 年的情况，故将本次调查称为 2011 年全国慢性病防控能力调查。

本报告主体包括三章。第一章为绪论，阐述了调查背景、调查目的、调查内容与方法、数据采集方式、职责分工、质量控制、数据清理与分析方法等。第二章为分析结果，主要分为九个部分，包括数据完成情况、慢性病防控政策能力、慢性病防控基础配置能力、慢性病防控教育培训与指导能力、慢性病防控合作与参与能力、慢性病监测能力、慢性病干预与管理能力、慢性病评估能力和慢性病科研能力。第三章为主要发现和建议，根据本次调查结果，结合前两次调查内容，阐述主要发现并提出政策建议。

本次调查得到了全国 31 个省（自治区、直辖市）和新疆生产建设兵团卫生行政部门、疾病预防控制中心及被调查基层医疗卫生机构的大力支持，在此对所有参与调查的人员表示由衷的感谢。

限于编者水平，书中难免有不足之处，敬请各位读者不吝赐教。

主 编

2015 年 10 月

摘 要

一、调查目的

系统评估2011年我国慢性病防控能力现状及慢性病防控能力建设中的制约因素和需求情况；并与2009年调查结果作对比，了解我国慢性病防控能力变化情况；综合评估各省慢性病防控能力；为落实国家基本公共卫生服务项目提供基线数据，为加强我国慢性病防控能力建设、制定慢性病防控相关政策提供依据。

二、内容与方法

采用中国疾控中心开发的全国慢性病防控能力在线调查系统，于2012年8月至2013年3月，对全国31个省（自治区、直辖市）和新疆生产建设兵团的省级、地市级和县（区）级疾病预防控制中心和随机抽样的3000家基层医疗卫生机构进行调查。调查内容包括各级慢性病防控政策能力、慢性病防控基础配置能力、教育培训与指导能力、合作与参与能力、监测能力、干预与管理能力、评估能力和科研能力等。各级疾控中心负责本级疾控中心调查表的在线填报，县（区）级疾控中心还承担对辖区内基层医疗卫生机构的调查及调查表在线填报。

三、主要结果

本次应调查全国3340家疾控中心，包括省级32家、地市级347家、县（区）级2961家及3000家基层医疗卫生机构（包括1500家社区卫生服务中心和1500家乡镇卫生院）。在线调查结束时，共有32家省级疾控中心、346家地市级疾控中心、2937家县（区）级疾控中心和2955家基层医疗卫生机构填写了调查问卷，应答率分别为100%、99.7%、99.2%和98.5%。调查主要结果如下：

（一）慢性病防控政策能力

反映各级政府或卫生行政部门对慢性病防控工作的认识程度和给予相关支持，主要包括政策认定能力、政策制定能力、政策执行能力、政策评估能力和政策调整能力等。考虑到数据的可获得性和实际意义等，本报告仅针对各地、各级慢性病防控的政策认定能力和政策制定能力进行分析、评价。

1. 政策认定能力

政策认定能力，即将社会问题转化为政策问题的能力。本调查中主要包括，财政经费支持情况、政府领导参与情况和政策倡导情况等三个方面。2011年，全国84.4%的省级政府财政经费配置了慢性病防控专项经费，地市级和县（区）级的比例分别为28.0%和

21.5%。各地政府财政配置慢性病防控专项经费的比例，东部地区（34.1%）高于中部（19.0%）和西部地区（17.1%）。

省、地市、县（区）级政府领导参与慢性病防控相关活动的比例分别为 46.9%、40.8%和 36.1%。

2011 年，各级、各地人大会议或政协会议（简称两会）上，提有慢性病防控为主题的议案或提案的比例按省（43.8%）、地市（17.9%）、县（区）（5.9%）逐级递减。其中省级两会慢性病防控相关提案或议案平均 10 个，地市级平均 2.2 个，县（区）级平均 2.4 个。

2. 政策制定能力

政策制定能力主要以所在地区本级政府或卫生行政部门制定并发布现行慢性病防控相关规划的情况为衡量。2011 年，全国有 7 个省（自治区、直辖市），38 个地市和 432 个县（区）颁布慢性病防控相关规划，所占比例分别为 21.9%、11.0%和 14.7%；全国有 26 个省级（81.3%）、106 个地市（30.6%）和 753 个县（区）（25.6%）有现行的慢性病防控相关工作（实施）方案。

（二）慢性病防控基础配置能力

主要包括部门、人员、经费、设备等的配置情况。

1. 部门设置

2011 年，全国省级疾控中心均设有承担慢性病防控工作的部门，地市级和县（区）级的设置比例分别为 93.4%和 89.2%（2009 年分别为 90.5%和 79.3%）。从地区分布来看，东、中、西部地区设有承担慢性病防控工作部门的比例分别为 95.5%、94.8%和 81.7%。

全国省级疾控中心内设立专门承担慢性病防控工作部门的比例为 78.1%，地市级和县（区）级疾控中心设立专门部门的比例明显降低，分别为 36.4%和 14.8%，但较 2009 年有所提高［2009 年地市和县（区）两级比例分别为 27.2%和 7.1%］。

2. 人力资源配置

2011 年，全国省及以下各级疾控中心慢性病防控在岗总人数为 9315 人，较 2009 年（8263 人）和 2008 年（7483 人）调查时有所增长。三级平均配置人数分别为 10.8 人、4.1 人和 2.8 人，与 2009 年调查数据相比，省级有所下降，地市级有所上升、县（区）级持平（2009 年三级分别为 11.8 人、3.9 人和 2.8 人）。2011 年，全国省及以下各级疾控中心专职慢性病防控人员总数为 6370 人，省、地市、县（区）三级分别为 310 人、910 人和 4150 人。专职人员占慢性病防控在岗人员的 68.4%，占疾控中心总在岗人数的 3.2%，较 2008 年（4796 人，2.6%）和 2009 年（3656 人，1.9%）均有所增加。在应答的 2955 家基层医疗卫生机构中，平均在岗卫生技术人员数 39.8 人，社区卫生服务中心和乡镇卫生院平均分别为 49.4 人和 30.3 人。

调查显示，各级疾控中心慢性病防控在岗人员平均年龄为 38.4 岁，省级、地市级和县（区）级差别不大，分别为38.1岁、40.0岁和38.1岁。全国范围内，35~44岁组人员所占比例最高，为35.1%。各级疾控中心慢性病防控在岗人员的平均工作年限为4.7年，其中省级人员平均工作年限最长，为7.4年，地市级和县（区）级分别为5.8年和4.4年。

我国慢性病防控人员队伍的学历水平和专业素质都比较高。全国慢性病防控在岗人员中具有本科以上学历的比例为43.7%，较2009年调查时（38.2%）有所增长。省、地市、县（区）三级呈现逐级下降趋势，分别为88.6%、64.1%和37.9%。各级疾控中心慢性病防控在岗人员中有医学专业背景的比例为89.9%，其中预防医学或公共卫生、临床医学为主要专业，分别占40.1%和30.1%，均较2009年（41.3%和33%）有所下降。省、地市、县（区）三级疾控中心中具有预防医学或公共卫生专业的人员比例分别为69.8%、50.4%和36.9%。应答的9266名慢性病防控在岗人员中7150名（77.2%）取得执业资格，省、地市和县（区）三级分别为85.5%、85.6%和75.2%。全国慢性病防控工作人员中具有初级职称的比例最高为38.9%，具有中级职称的占36.6%，具有副高级职称的占8.7%，具有正高级职称的占2.3%。

3. 经费配置能力

经费配置能力主要指被调查疾控中心2011年到账的慢性病防控工作经费情况、被调查基层医疗卫生机构2011年到账的基本公共卫生服务经费情况。2011年，全国57.3%的疾控中心配置了慢性病防控工作经费，其中省、地市、县（区）三级该比例分别为96.9%、76.0%和54.6%。省级疾控中心慢性病防控工作经费平均为181.6万元，地市级和县（区）级分别为17.0万元和13.7万元；与2009年的各级经费配置额度相比［省、地市和县（区）分别为147.7、14.2和9.1万元］有一定幅度提高。全国各地各级疾控中心的慢性病防控工作经费占疾控中心业务经费比例为4.4%，较2009年（2.7%）有所增长。省、地市和县（区）三级分别为2.0%、3.1%和7.4%。

在应答的2955家基层医疗卫生机构中，有2822家在2011年获得了基本公共卫生服务经费，占95.5%；获得基本公共卫生服务经费的平均数额为85.4万元，其中乡镇卫生院平均数额为52.4万元，社区卫生服务中心平均数额为117.9万元。2011年，在获得基本公共卫生服务经费的2822家基层医疗卫生机构中，34.8%的财政拨款来源于基本公共卫生服务经费，较2009年有所下降（37.6%）；其中乡镇卫生院为36.3%，社区卫生服务中心为34.1%。

4. 设备配置能力

本部分主要调查了基层医疗卫生机构的基本设备配备情况，调查发现，基层医疗卫生机构配备体重秤、身高计、腰围尺、血压计、血糖仪的比例均在90%以上，其次为心电图机（82.8%）、B超（79.5%）、生化仪（72.1%）、健教设备（71.9%）和X线机（66.8%），配备肺功能仪的比例最低，仅为16.3%。

（三）慢性病防控教育培训与指导能力

本部分主要包括培训能力、指导能力和知识普及能力。培训能力包括组织培训和参与培训，指导能力即对下级机构开展慢性病防控工作现场指导的情况，知识普及能力指基层医疗卫生机构向大众宣传慢性病防控相关知识的情况。

1. 培训能力

2011 年全国各级疾控中心有 2227 家机构举办过各类慢性病防控相关培训班，比例为 67. 2%，（2009 年为 43. 5%），其中东部、中部、西部地区各级疾控中心举办各类相关培训的比例分别为 79. 8%、63. 5%、60. 5%，省级、地市级、县（区）级疾控中心举办各类相关培训的比例分别为 100. 0%、70. 5%、66. 4%。

全国省级、地市级、县（区）级疾控中心均以举办本级慢性病防控相关培训班的比例最高，分别为 93. 8%、63. 9%、65. 6%。全国各级慢性病防控相关培训班共培训 298 273人次。全国各级慢性病防控培训中，以县（区）级培训人次数最多，占总培训人次数的 95. 3%。

各级疾控中心均以举办本级继续教育培训为主，其中 22 个省级疾控中心、91 个地市级疾控中心举办了本级的继续教育培训。全国各级慢性病防控相关继续教育培训班共培训 38 995 人次，其中由县（区）级疾控中心举办的培训班培训人次数最多，占总培训人次数的 90. 8%。

本次调查共有 2437 个基层医疗卫生机构应答举办了慢性病防控相关培训班，占被调查基层医疗卫生机构的 82. 5%（2009 年为 58. 8%），其中社区卫生服务中心 1200 家，占被调查同类机构的 81. 2%（2009 年为 72. 5%），乡镇卫生院 1237 个，占被调查同类机构的 83. 8%（2009 年为 44. 6%）。

2. 技术指导能力

全国有 30 个省级疾控中心开展过对县（区）级疾控中心的现场指导工作，比例为 93. 8%（2009 年为 100%），85. 5%的地市级疾控中心指导过县（区）级疾控中心（2009 年为 64. 7%），79. 5%的县（区）级疾控中心开展过对基层医疗卫生机构的指导工作（2009 年为 48. 3%）。

全国有 2160 个基层医疗卫生机构对辖区内的社区卫生服务站/村卫生室开展过慢性病现场技术指导，占被调查机构的比例为 73. 1%（2009 年为 49. 0%），其中乡镇卫生院 1220 个，比例为 82. 6%（2009 年为 36. 9%）、社区卫生服务中心 940 个，比例为 63. 6%（2009 年为 60. 8%）。

3. 知识普及能力

2011 年，被调查基层医疗卫生机构在高血压日开展活动的机构比例达 91. 0%，较 2009 年（56. 3%）有大幅度增长，其中社区卫生服务中心为 96. 5%、乡镇卫生院为 85. 4%。在世界无烟日、世界糖尿病日、全民健康生活方式日、世界脑卒中日和世界心脏病日开展过相关宣传活动的机构比例依次降低，分别为88.5%、87.8%、68.2%、48.5%和41.8%。

（四）慢性病防控合作与参与能力

慢性病防控合作与参与能力是一个广义的概念，它包括与其他机构或部门在慢性病防控领域开展项目合作的能力和参与上级机构慢性病防控相关工作的能力。

1. 合作能力

2011年，36.2%的疾控中心与媒体开展过合作，居首位，且高于2009年的20.2%。与独立健康教育机构、专业防办、二级及以上医院和NGO等其他机构合作的比例分别为13.6%、6.1%、28.2%和5.9%。省级、地市级、县（区）级疾控中心开展慢性病防控相关合作的比例逐渐降低。

2. 参与能力

省级、地市级、县（区）级疾控中心参与本级卫生行政部门政策制定的比例分别为59.4%、30.9%和29.1%；参与本级卫生以外其他行政部门慢性病防控工作的比例，省级、地市级、县（区）级分别为62.5%、34.4%和29.7%；参与上级卫生行政部门或业务机构慢性病防控工作的比例，省级、地市级、县（区）级分别为71.9%、28.6%和18.0%。

被调查基层医疗卫生机构参与慢性病防控相关项目或科研工作的比例为12.4%，其中乡镇卫生院为7.1%，社区卫生服务中心为17.7%。参与国家级慢性病防控相关项目或科研工作的比例为4.8%；参与省级、地市级和县（区）级慢性病防控相关项目或科研工作的比例分别为2.9%、3.2%和5.5%。

（五）慢性病监测能力

1. 死因监测

2011年，全国有66.1%的疾控中心开展了死因监测工作。省级、地市级、县（区）级疾控中心开展此项工作的比例分别为96.9%、80.1%和63.4%。2011年开展死因监测的任务来源主要是上级，占93.3%，来源于本级的比例为32.4%，来源于国际级的比例仅为2.5%。在开展死因监测的地区中，开展覆盖所有县（区）死因监测的省和地市比例分别为48.4%和79.4%；开展死因监测工作覆盖所有街道和乡镇的县（区）级比例为84.3%。死因监测数据发布或利用的首要形式是编写年报，省级、地市级和县（区）级编写年报的机构比例分别为90.3%、64.3%、57.4%。各地、各级疾控中心所在地开展死因监测中信息被采纳的比例为54.8%，省级（80.6%）比例高于地市（62.8%）和县（区）级（53.2%）。

57.6%的被调查基层医疗卫生机构开展了死亡病例报告工作。其中，乡镇卫生院为47.2%，社区卫生服务中心为68.1%，均高于2009年。东、中、西部地区开展死亡病例报告的机构所占的比例分别为74.2%、51.3%和44.0%。

2. 慢性病危险因素监测

2011年，省级疾控中心所在地区开展各类慢性病危险因素监测（除血脂）的机构比例均大于90%，且均明显高于地市级和县（区）级。各级疾控中心所在地区开展各类危险因素监测的任务来源主要是上级机构，其次是本级。数据信息发布及利用的首要方式为编写年报，随后依次是发表论文、出版报告和媒体发布。

3. 发病和患病登记/报告

恶性肿瘤、脑卒中和心肌梗死的病例报告工作在省级、地市级和县（区）级疾控中心开展的比例依次降低，其中省级开展恶性肿瘤登记的比例最高，为 90.6%；县（区）级开展心肌梗死报告的比例最低，为 20.6%。东部地区开展比例高于中、西部地区，其中东部地区开展恶性肿瘤登记的比例最高，为 34.4%；西部地区开展心肌梗死报告的比例最低，为 14.2%。各级疾控中心开展覆盖所有县（区）/街道和乡镇的恶性肿瘤、脑卒中与心肌梗死病例报告的比例分别为 82.2%、86.3%、87.7%。发病信息的主要发布形式为编写年报，其中恶性肿瘤病例报告中利用此形式发布数据的比例占 61.1%，脑卒中和心肌梗死病例报告的比例分别为 60.4%和 60.4%。

共有 27.1%（2009 年为 18.6%）的被调查基层医疗卫生机构开展了新发脑卒中病例报告工作，其中乡镇卫生院开展比例为 17.4%，社区卫生服务中心的开展比例为 36.9%。开展急性心肌梗死病例报告的基层医疗机构占 23.8%（2009 年为 13.0%），其中乡镇卫生院开展比例为 15.1%，社区卫生服务中心的开展比例为 32.5%。

（六）慢性病干预与管理能力

1. 主要慢性病及其危险因素干预

2011 年，各级疾控中心开展或参与了慢性病高危人群个体化干预的比例为 28.1%，较 2009 年有所上升（13.7%），分别为高血压 64.1%、糖尿病 62.8%、恶性肿瘤 21.4%、脑卒中 15.1%、冠心病 14.3%和慢性呼吸系统疾病 8.7%，较 2009 年均有提高（2009 年分别为 36.1%、32.2%、16.1%、10.9%、11.0%、6.5%）。

2011 年全国分别有 35.2%、24.7%、20.7%、16.2%的疾控中心开展了烟草使用、膳食、身体活动、酒精使用的相关干预项目或工作，较 2009 年开展这四项干预工作的比例明显升高（烟草使用 18.4%、膳食 15.4%、身体活动 12.2%、酒精使用 9.3%）。2011 年全国分别有 20.2%、33.4%、31.8%、16.2%的疾控中心开展了超重肥胖、高血压、高血糖、血脂异常相关的干预项目或工作，较 2009 年开展这四项干预工作的比例明显升高（2009 年分别是 11.5%、19.9%、17.2%与 9.9%）。

2. 慢性病患者及高危人群早发现

2011 年，94.1%的基层医疗卫生机构开展了 35 岁以上居民首诊测血压工作，其中 96.5%的社区卫生服务中心和 91.7%的乡镇卫生院开展了 35 岁以上居民首诊测血压工作，均比 2009 年明显提高（2009 年分别是 89.1%与 43.8%）。

2011 年，90.9%的社区卫生服务中心和 93.4%的乡镇卫生院开展了 65 岁以上老年人免费健康体检工作，比 2009 年（分别是 74.8%与 45.0%）明显上升。在开展此项工作的基层医疗卫生机构中，各项检查项目开展比例从高到低依次为，血压（99.9%）、体重

(98.8%)、身高 (98.7%)、血糖 (95.5%)、腰围 (93.0%)、心电图检查 (80.9%)、血脂 (64.9%)、X 线检查 (36.6%)。

3. 主要慢性病患者和高危人群管理

2011 年，96.8%的被调查基层医疗卫生机构开展了高血压患者建档工作，明显高于 2009 年 (62.8%)。44.0%的被调查基层医疗卫生机构开展了血压正常高值者建档工作，明显高于 2009 年 (26.8%)。在被调查基层医疗卫生服务机构中，分别有 96.0%和 34.3%开展了高血压患者随访管理和血压正常高值者随访管理。经估算，开展高血压患者管理的基层医疗卫生机构所在辖区内，高血压患者的管理率为 14.2%，管理人群规范管理率为 82.6%，控制率为 53.1% (均比 2009 年调查数据有所提高，2009 年三者分别为 12.0%、73.8%和 48.7%)。

2011 年，95.6%的被调查基层医疗卫生机构开展了糖尿病患者建档工作，28.2%的被调查基层医疗卫生机构开展了糖尿病高危人群即空腹血糖受损/糖耐量减低者建档工作，这两项工作的开展比例均较 2009 年有所提高，2009 年分别为 61.3%和 15.5%。在被调查基层医疗卫生服务机构中，分别有 94.7%和 23.9%开展了糖尿病患者随访管理与空腹血糖受损/糖耐量减低者随访管理。经估算，开展糖尿病患者管理的基层医疗卫生机构所在辖区内，糖尿病患者管理率为 10.1%，管理人群规范管理率为 82.5%，控制率为 51.7% (2009 年，管理率、规范管理率和控制率分别为 7.9%、80.1%和 50.0%)。

4. 慢性病康复服务能力

2011 年，676 个被调查基层卫生机构提供脑卒中患者机械康复服务，占 22.9%，社区卫生服务中心和乡镇卫生院开展脑卒中患者康复工作的比例分别为 38.6%和 7.1%。

(七) 慢性病评估能力

2011 年全国有 30.6%的卫生行政部门或疾控中心对本辖区慢性病应对情况开展定期评估，比 2009 年的比例 (13.3%) 明显增高，省级的比例为 37.5%，比 2009 年 (40.6%) 略有下降，但高于地市级 (29.8%) 与县 (区) 级 (30.6%)，地市级与县 (区) 级开展定期评估的比例比 2009 年 (19.7%和 12.2%) 明显增加。

2011 年全国各级疾控中心参与本辖区基层医疗卫生机构考核或评估的比例为 71.1%，明显高于 2009 年的比例 (40.9%)，省级、地市级与县 (区) 级疾控中心参与本辖区基层医疗卫生机构考核或评估的比例分别为 71.9%、70.8%和 71.2%，均高于 2009 年各级疾控中心参与的比例 (62.5%、45.1%、40.2%)。

(八) 慢性病科研能力

2011 年，全国 6.7%的疾控中心主持或参与了慢性病领域国内课题，略高于 2009 年 (6.1%) 的调查结果。2011 年，全国仅有 1.1%的疾控中心参与国际科研课题，低于 2009 年的调查结果 (3.8%)。2011 年，全国仅有 8.3%的疾控中心有工作人员在国内外期刊发表过论文，略低于 2009 年的比例 (9.7%)。2011 年，全国仅有 27 个疾控中心的工作人员出版过慢性病方面专著，所占比例是0.8%，低于2009年的比例（4.8%）。2011年，全国获科技进步奖的疾控中心有27个，占0.8%。省、地市、县（区）三级机构所占比例依次降低，分别为12.5%、3.8%和0.3%［2009年，省、地市和县（区）级的比例分别为12.5%、5.8%和2.7%］。

（九）慢性病防控综合能力

本次综合评估是从之前评估的8个模块中选取核心指标，分别是政策能力模块中的3个指标，包括指标1政府慢性病防控专项财政经费配置情况、指标2有以慢性病防控为主题的提案或议案的情况、指标3制定慢性病综合规划（政府或多部门制定）的情况；基础配置能力模块的3个指标，包括指标4专门慢性病防控科所设置情况、指标5专职慢性病防控人员占疾控卫生技术人员比例、指标6基层医疗卫生机构同时配置血糖仪和血压计的情况；教育培训和指导能力模块的3个指标，包括指标7主办慢性病防控相关培训班情况、指标8县级疾控中心对基层医疗卫生机构开展指导的情况、指标9基层医疗卫生机构举办健康讲座的情况；合作模块的2个指标，包括指标10疾控中心与媒体合作的情况、指标11开展多部门合作的情况；早期发现与监测模块3个指标，包括指标12开展全人群死因监测的情况、指标13开展危险因素监测的情况、指标14基层医疗卫生机构开展35岁以上首诊测血压的情况；干预与管理能力模块4个指标，指标15开展全民健康生活方式行动的情况、指标16基层医疗卫生机构高血压患者血压控制情况、指标17基层医疗卫生机构糖尿病患者血糖控制情况、指标18基层医疗卫生机构同时开展高血压和糖尿病患者双向转诊的情况；评估能力模块1个指标，指标19疾控中心参与基层医疗卫生机构考核或评估的情况；科研能力模块1个指标，指标20疾控中心慢性病防控人员人均发表论文的情况。共20个核心指标建立慢性病防控能力综合评估指标体系，每个指标赋值5分，共100分。根据各省（自治区、直辖市）和新疆生产建设兵团各指标完成情况，对各省（自治区、直辖市）新疆生产建设兵团慢性病防控综合能力进行评分并排序

四、主要发现

1. 2011年，全国慢性病防控政策能力已较2009年调查时有所提高，但仍然比较薄弱，各级各地政府对慢性病防控工作的重视程度有待提高，各地慢性病防控工作仍缺乏有力的政策保障。

2. 2011年，地市和县（区）级设置专门慢性病防控科所的比例较2009年均有一定幅度的提高。全国慢性病防控人员共9315人，较2009年和2008年分别增加1052人和1832人，占疾控中心总在岗人数的比例（4.6%）也呈上升趋势（2009年4.2%、2008年4.0%）；2011年慢性病防控队伍素质进一步提高，本科以上学历的慢性病防控工作人员占43.7%（2009年和2008年分别为38.2%、34.7%）。2011年，全国配置慢性病防控工作经费的疾控中心比例为57.3%，比2009年的比例（40.2%）有所提高；不同级别和地区疾控中心经费配备数额相差悬殊；慢性病防控工作经费占疾控中心业务经费比例为4.4%，较

2009 年（2.7%）有所增长。2011 年，在被调查基层医疗卫生服务机构中，乡镇卫生院配备各类慢性病防控相关设备的比例与 2009 年相比，已有大幅度增加，但除 X 线机外，仍低于社区卫生服务中心的各项设备配备比例。

3. 2011 年全国各级疾控中心举办过慢性病相关培训的比例为 67.2%，比 2009 年上升了 23.7 个百分点。2011 年全国各级疾控中心派人员参加慢性病防控相关培训的比例为 78.5%，比 2009 年上升了 24.7 个百分点。2011 年各级疾控中心对各项技能培训的需求均较高，应根据各级疾控中心具体需求情况开展有针对性的培训才能达到事半功倍的效果。乡镇卫生院开展慢性病防控相关各项活动的比例均低于社区卫生服务中心，乡镇卫生院知识普及的能力低于社区卫生服务中心。

4. 2011 年各级疾控中心与其他部门在慢性病防控方面的合作程度比 2009 年有所提高，但比例仍不高，特别是县（区）级疾控中心与其他机构开展合作的比例较低。2011 年，在慢性病防控工作中，主要合作机构仍然是媒体和二级及以上医院，合作比例明显高于其他机构。2011 年各级疾控中心与各类慢性病防控机构的合作比例均呈现省、地市、县（区）和东、中、西部下降趋势，与 2009 年的趋势一致。

5. 各类慢性病相关监测的开展比例整体偏低，特别是基层机构的监测水平亟待提高。在开展的各类慢性病相关监测中，地方代表性较好，其中覆盖所有县（区）/街道和乡镇的比例均在 50%以上，能更好地反映被监测地区的实际情况。2011 年，在开展的各类慢性病相关监测中，编写年报仍然是信息发布及利用的主要形式。

6. 2011 年，各级疾控中心开展主要慢性病及其危险因素干预工作的比例较 2009 年有所提高，但整体水平仍然较低。35 岁以上居民首诊测血压制度和为 65 岁以上老年人免费健康体检制度在基层医疗卫生机构中已初步建立，乡镇卫生院早期发现的能力与 2009 年相比有大幅度提高。基层医疗卫生机构承担高血压、糖尿病患者管理工作的比例较 2009 年有较大幅度的提高，辖区管理率虽有提高，但相对庞大的患者人群仍显不足，规范化管理过程和管理效果仍需提高。高危人群管理工作较 2009 年有一定程度改善，但仍处于较低水平。

7. 2011 年，地市和县（区）级疾控中心或卫生行政部门对本辖区慢性病应对情况的评估能力较 2009 年有所加强。各级疾控中心参与本辖区基层医疗卫生机构考核评估的比例较高，超过了 70%，较 2009 年的比例明显提高，省、地市、县（区）各级均有不同程度的提高。

8. 省级疾控中心相对具有较强的慢性病科研能力，明显高于地市和县（区）级疾控中心；东部地区疾控中心的科研能力高于中、西部地区。但从全国总体水平来看，全国疾控中心慢性病防控方面的科研能力仍然较为薄弱。

五、政策建议

1. 加强政策倡导，均衡区域发展。
2. 稳步提升慢性病防控基础配置。
3. 发挥省级技术培训和指导能力优势，提高基层慢性病防治的工作能力。
4. 加强多部门的合作，提高慢性病防控决策参与能力。
5. 抓好慢性病防控基础性工作，确保工作质量。
6. 提高各级疾控中心对慢性病应对情况的评估能力，积极开展科学合作。

Abstract

1. Objectives

1.1 Systematically assessing the status quo of the capacity for the prevention and control of noncommunicable diseases (NCDs) in China in 2011 and restricts and needs in construction of national capacity for the prevention and control of NCDs.

1.2 Knowing about the change of country's capacity for NCDs' prevention and control compared with the findings of 2009.

1.3 Comprehensively assessing the capacity for the prevention and control of NCDs in every province.

1.4 Providing baseline data to carry out national basic public health service projects and basis for strengthening the capacity construction of the prevention and control of NCDs; moreover, laying down relevant policies on prevention and control of NCDs in China.

2. Content and methods

This survey was conducted from August 2012 through March 2013 over the Centers for Disease Control and Prevention (CDCs) at the provincial, municipal and county/district levels across 31 provinces/autonomous regions/municipalities directly under the central government and Xinjiang Production and Construction Corps and 3000 primary health care units (PHCUs) by using the online survey system on national capacity for the prevention and control of NCDs developed by Chinese Center for Disease Prevention and Control. The contents of the survey include the capacity of the prevention and control of NCDs refers to policy in each administrative area, basic deployment, educational training and direction, cooperation and participation, surveillance capacity, intervention and management capacity, assessment capacity and scientific research capacity, and so on. Each-level CDCs were responsible for online filing of survey forms within their respective jurisdiction, and the county-level CDCs were also responsible for carrying out a survey on PHCUs within their jurisdiction and the online filing of survey forms.

3. Main Results

This survey involved 3340 CDCs (including 32 ones at the provincial level, 347 ones at the municipal level and 2961 ones at the county/district level) and 3000 PHCUs (1500 community health centers and 1500 town public health centers). At the end of the online survey, 32 provincial

CDCs, 346 municipal CDCs, 2937 county/district CDCs and 2955 PHCUs filed in the questionnaire in total. The response rates were respectively 100%, 99. 7%, 99. 2% and 98. 5%. The overall response rate in this survey was 99. 3%, higher than 2009 (97. 2%). The main results of the survey are as follows.

3. 1 Capacity on policies for the prevention and control of NCDs

This capacity can reflect on each administrative level of governments or health administrations' awareness of and support for the work of prevention and control of NCDs, including the capacity for making, executing, assessing and adjusting policies, etc. Considering the availability and actual meaning of data, this report only analyzes and evaluates the capacity for policy making and laying down policies on the prevention and control of NCDs at each locality and level.

3. 1. 1 Capacity for policy making

Capacity for policy making means the capability of transforming social issues into policies. This survey mainly involves the following three aspects: support by financial funds, leadership and participation by governments and policy advocacy. In 2011, 84. 4% of the provincial financial funds in China allocated special funds for NCDs prevention and control, which at the municipal and county/district levels were 28. 0% and 21. 5%. The rate was 34. 1% in the eastern region, higher than 19. 0% in the middle region and 17. 1% in the western region.

The proportion of participation in the prevention and control of NCDs by government leaders of the provincial, municipal and county levels were 46. 9%, 40. 8% and 36. 1%, respectively.

In 2011, at the people's congress conferences or political consultative conferences ("Two Sessions") of each level and locality, the rates of proposals or bills with the subject of prevention and control of NCDs decreased level by level: 43. 8% at the provincial level, followed by 17. 9% at the municipal level and 5. 9% at the county/district level. On average, the number of proposals or bills at Two Sessions at the provincial level was 10, 2. 2 at the municipal level and 2. 4 at the county/district level.

3. 1. 2 Capacity for laying down policies

The capacity for laying down policies was mainly measured by the status quo on a certain local government or health administration laying down and enacting current plan on the prevention and control of NCDs. In 2011, 7 provinces/municipalities directly under the central government/autonomous regions, 38 cities at the municipal level and 432 counties/districts enacted relevant plans on the prevention and control of NCDs, accounting for 21. 9%, 11. 0% and 14. 7%, respectively. 26 provinces (81. 3%), 106 cities at the municipal level (30. 6%) and 753 counties/districts (25. 6%) have had in place current plans (for implementation) on the prevention and control of NCDs.

3.2 Capacity for basic deployment of the prevention and control of NCDs

Mainly including the deployment of department, personnel, funds, equipment, and so on.

3.2.1 Deployment of departments

Up to 2011, all China provincial CDCs have established departments responsibled for the prevention and control of NCDs. The rates of deployment of such departments at the municipal and county/district levels were 93.4% and 89.2% (the rates were respectively 90.5% and 79.3% in 2009). In terms of regional distribution, such rates were 95.5%, 94.8% and 81.7% in the eastern, middle and western regions.

The proportion of the departments which particularly responsible for the prevention and control of NCDs established in the provincial CDCs in China was 78.1%. The proportion apparently declined at the municipal and county/district levels, which were separately 36.4% and 14.8%, however, higher than that in 2009 (27.2% and 7.1%).

3.2.2 Deployment of human resources

In 2011, the personnel in service engaged in the prevention and control of NCDs at CDCs at and below the provincial level in China was totally 9315, which saw an increase compared to 8263 in 2009 and 7483 in 2008. The average numbers of deployed personnel at three levels were respectively 10.8, 4.1 and 2.8. To be specific, in comparison to 2009, there was a descent at the provincial level, an increase at the municipal level and no fluctuation at the county/district level (respectively 11.8, 3.9 and 2.8 in 2009). In 2011, the number of full-time personnel for the prevention and control of NCDs at and below the provincial level of CDCs was totally 6370, among whom 310910 and 4150 employees work at the provincial, municipal and county/district levels. Full-time personnel accounted for 68.4% in all employees working for the cause of preventing and controlling NCDs and 3.2% of total workers at CDCs, which both faced an increase compared with those of 2008 (4796, 2.6%) and 2009 (3656, 1.9%). In the 2955 responded PHCUs, technical personnel in service was 39.8 on average and such numbers for community health centers and town public health centers were respectively 49.4 and 30.3.

According to the survey, the average age of personnel in service at each-level CDCs was 38.4. There are no remarkable differences among the provincial, municipal and county/district levels, 38.1, 40.0 and 38.1, respectively. Nationwide, the group of 35 ~ 44 accounted for the highest proportion, 35.1%. The average work seniority of the personnel in service at NCD posts of each-level CDCs was 4.7 years, personnel working at the provincial level featured the longest work seniority on average: 7.4 years, while those at the municipal and county/district levels worked for a less longer time period: 5.8 and 4.4 years, respectively.

The team of NCD personnel in China featured a high academic level and professional quality. 43. 7% of the personnel in service for the cause of preventing and controlling NCDs in China have a bachelor's degree or above, with a growth compared with that of 2009 (38. 2%). This proportion decreased level by level from the provincial level to the municipal and county/district levels: 88. 6%, 64. 1% and 37. 9% orderly. 89. 9% of the personnel in service working for the prevention and control of NCDs at each level of CDCs have the background of medical specialty, mainly are preventive medicine (40. 1%) and clinical medicine (30. 1%), which decreasd compared with 2009 (41. 3% and 33%, respectively). The personnel with the major of preventive medicine or clinical medicine at the CDCs of provincial, municipal and county/district level accounted for 69. 8%, 50. 4% and 26. 4%, respectively. 7150 out of 9266 employees in service for the prevention and control of NCDs (77. 2%) have obtained the practice qualification - the proportion at the three levels of province, municipality and county/district was 85. 5%, 85. 6% and 75. 2%. Those with primary title working for the prevention and control of NCDs national wide accounted for 38. 9%, with intermediate title was 36. 6%, 8. 7% with sub-senior title and 2. 3% in senior title.

3. 2. 3 Capacity for deploying funds

The capacity for deploying funds mainly refers to the funds credited to surveyed CDCs in 2011 for the work of disease prevention and control and basic public health service funds credited to surveyed PHCUs in 2011. Up to 2011, 57. 3% of CDCs nationwide had deployed funds for the prevention and control of NCDs. The proportion for the three levels of province, municipality and county/district was 96. 9%, 76. 0% and 54. 6% in order. The average funds for provincial CDCs were RMB 1. 816 million, and RMB 0. 17 million and RMB 0. 137 million at the municipal and county/district levels, which experienced a certain extent of increase compared with the funds in 2009 (RMB 1. 477 million, RMB 0. 142 million and RMB 0. 091 million respectively at the provincial, municipal and county/district levels). The funds for the prevention and control of NCDs at each-level CDCs in China accounted for 4. 4% in the funds for the business of disease prevention and control, a rising compared with 2009 (2. 7%). This proportion at the three levels of province, municipality and county/district was respectively 2. 0%, 3. 1% and 7. 4%.

Among the 2955 PHCUs, 2822 have been allocated funds for basic public health services, accounting for 95. 5%. The average amount of basic public health service funds was RMB 0. 854 million, among which RMB 0. 524 million was allocated to town public health centers and RMB 1. 179 million to community health centers. In 2011, among the 2822 PHCUs that obtained funds for basic public health services, 34. 8% of the fiscal appropriations derive from the funds for basic public health services, which saw a decline compared with 2009 (37. 6%), among which town public health centers accounted for 36. 3% and community health centers was 34. 1%.

3. 2. 4 Capacity for deploying equipment

This section mainly focuses on basic information on equipment deployment at PHCUs. It is found that over 90% of the PHCUs were equipped with weighing scales, height scales, waist circumference rulers, sphygmomanometers, glucose meters; 82.8% with electrocardiographs, 79.5% with B ultrasonic instruments; 72.1% with biochemical instruments; 71.9% with fitness equipment; 66.8% with X-ray machines; only 16.3% with lung function meters.

3.3 Educational training and direction capacity for the prevention and control of NCDs

This section mainly includes training capacity, direction capacity and knowledge popularization capacity. Training capacity includes organizing and participating in training. Direction capacity means an institution of the lower level conducting on-site direction over the prevention and control of NCDs. Knowledge popularization capacity expresses publicizing knowledge relevant to the prevention and control of NCDs by basic-level medical health servicc institutions.

3.3.1 Training capacity

In 2011, 2227 CDCs (67.2%, 43.5% in 2009) of each level countrywide held all kinds of workshops related to the prevention and control of NCDs. The proportion of workshops in the eastern, middle and western regions was 79.8%, 63.5%, 60.5% orderly, and was 100.0%, 70.5% and 66.4% at the provincial, municipal and county/district levels .

The CDCs of the provincial, municipal and county/district levels accounted for the highest proportion at the level of their own jurisdiction, which was separatelg 93.8%, 63.9% and 65.6%. Altogether 298 273 people have been trained at relevant workshops of the prevention and control of NCDs at each level. Among the trainings countrywide related to the prevention and control of NCDs, people at the county/district level accounted for the highest proportion, 95.3% of the overall trained personnel.

Each-level CDCs were mainly responsible for holding continuous education and training, among which 22 provincial CDCs and 91 municipal ones hold the continuous education and training of their corresponding level. Altogether 38 995 people got trained at each level workshops for continuous education and training related to the prevention and control of NCDs, among whom personnel getting trained at CDCs of the county/district level accounted for the highest proportion, 90.8% of the overall trained personnel.

In this survey, 2 437 PHCUs (82.5%) (58.8% in 2009) in total have held CDC related workshops. 1 200 were community health centers, accounting for 81.2% in the surveyed institutions of the same kind (72.5% in 2009), and 1237 were town public health centers, making up 83.8% in the surveyed institutions of the same kind (44.6% in 2009).

3.3.2 Technical direction capacity

30 provincial CDCs in China have ever carried out on-site direction work over the county/dis-

trict CDCs, accounting for 93. 8% (100% in 2009), 85. 5% of the municipal CDCs have done the same over the county/district CDCs (64. 7% in 2009), 79. 5% of the county/district CDCs have done the same over PHCUs (48. 3% in 2009).

There are 2160 PHCUs have conducted on-site technical direction on the prevention and control of NCDs over community health service stations/ village health centers, accounting for 73. 1% in surveyed institutions (49. 0% in 2009), among which 1220 units (82. 6%) were town public health centers (36. 9% in 2009), and 940 units (63. 6%) were community health centers (60. 8% in 2009).

3. 3. 3 Knowledge popularization capacity

In 2011, surveyed PHCUs occupied the highest proportion in carrying out activities on the "High Blood Pressure Day", reaching 91. 0%, which was a remarkable increase compared with 2009 (56. 3%), among which community health centers accounted for 96. 5% and town public health centers accounted for 85. 4%. 88. 5% of the PHCUs have organized relevant publicity activities on the "World No-Tobacco Day". This proportion declined on the "World Diabetes Day", the "World Hypertension Day", the "National Healthy Life Style Day", the "World Stroke Day" and the "World Heart Disease Day", which were 87. 8%, 68. 2%, 48. 5% and 41. 8%, respectively.

3. 4. Capacity for the collaboration of and participation in the prevention and control of NCDs

The capacity for the collaboration and participation in the prevention and control of NCDs is a concept in the broad sense. It comprises of the capability to cooperate with other institutions or departments on the prevention and control of NCDs and the capacity for participating in efforts for NCDs prevention and control led by institutions at higher levels.

3. 4. 1 Collaboration capacity

In 2011, 36. 2% of the CDCs had the experience of collaborating with mass media, higher than 2009 (20. 2%). This proportion was 13. 6%, 6. 1%, 28. 2% and 5. 9%, separately, with independent health educational institutions, professional prevention and control offices, hospitals of the 2nd level or above, NGOs and other institutions. The proportion of the CDCs at the provincial, municipal and county/district levels, which have engaged in efforts on the prevention and control of NCDs, decreased correspondingly in the order.

3. 4. 2 Participation capacity

The proportion of the participation by CDCs at the provincial, municipal and county/district levels in the efforts on the prevention and control of NCDs laid down by health administrations of the same level was respectively 59. 4%, 30. 9% and 29. 1%. The proportion of their participation in the efforts on the prevention and control of NCDs laid down by any other administrations other than health administrations of the same level was respectively 62. 5%, 34. 4% and 29. 7%. The proportion of their participation in the efforts on the prevention and control of NCDs laid down by any administrations of a higher level was respectively 71. 9%, 28. 6% and 18. 0%.

Among the surveyed PHCUs, 12. 4% units participated in programs or research activities of NCDs prevention and control among which 7. 1% were town public health centers and 17. 7% were community health centers. 4. 8% of them participated in programs or research activities funded by the national institutions, meanwhile, 2. 9%, 3. 2% and 5. 5%, separately participated in programs or research activities funded by the institutions at provincial, municipal and county/district levels.

3. 5. Capacity for surveillance of NCDs

3. 5. 1 Death cause surveillance

In 2011, 66. 1% CDCs monitored the death cause, to be specific, 96. 9% at provincial level, 80. 1% at municipal level, and 63. 4% at county/district level. To the source of tasks to carry out such surveillance in 2011, 93. 3% from the higher level, 32. 4% from the same level while only 2. 5% from the international level. Among the regions where death cause surveillance was carried out, 48. 4% of the provinces and 79. 4% of the municipalities have carried out such surveillance covering all counties/districts within their respective jurisdictions, while 84. 3% of the counties/districts have implemented such surveillance covering all streets and towns. The primary form of publishing or using death cause surveillance data is compiling an annual report. The proportion of the institutions which have compiled such report was: 90. 3% at the provincial level, 64. 3% at the municipal level, and 57. 4% at the county/district level. 54. 8% of the information collected through death cause surveillance carried out by the CDCs of each locality and level has been adopted, among which the proportion for the provincial level (80. 6%) was higher than the rest of the municipal level (62. 8%) and the county/district level (53. 2%).

57. 6% of the surveyed PHCUs have carried out death case report, among which town public health centers accounted for 47. 2% while community health service centers accounted for 68. 1%, both higher than that in 2009. 74. 2% of the institutions in the Eastern China, 51. 3% in the Central China, and 44. 0% in the Western China have implemented the death case reports.

3. 5. 2 Monitoring risk factors related to NCDs

In 2011, over 90% CDCs at the provincial level implemented various risk factor surveillance related to NCDs (blood lipids excluded), such proportion being remarkably higher than that at the municipal and county/district levels. The source of tasks to carry out such surveillance mainly come from the higher level and then the same level. The primary form of publishing or using death came surveillance data was compiling an annual report, then followed by publishing essays, publishing a report and publishing in the mass media.

3.5.3 Registration/report on incidence and prevalence

The proportion of reported cases of malignant tumor, stroke and MI (myocardial infarction) declined orderly at the levels of province, municipality and county/district. While as high as 90.6% of the CDCs at the provincial level implemented the activities of malignant tumor case reports, a few (20.6%) CDCs at the county level implemented the activities of MI case reports by contrast. 34.4% of the CDCs in the Eastern China implemented the activities of malignant tumor case reports, while fewer CDCs in Western China (14.2%) implemented the activities of MI case reports. The proportion of CDCs which have carried out reporting malignant tumor, stroke and MI cases covering all counties/districts/streets/towns was 82.2%, 86.3% and 87.7%. The results were mainly disseminated by publishing an annual report: 61.1% CDCs implemented the activities of malignant tumor case, 60.4% CDCs implemented the activities of stroke case and 60.4% CDCs implemented the activities of MI case reports have published reports.

As reported, 27.1% of the PHCUs implemented the activities of reporting new stroke case (18.6% in 2009), while 17.4% of town public health centers and 36.9% of community health centers also did. Approximately, 23.8% of PHCUs carried out acute MI case reporting (13.0% in 2009), while 15.1% of town public health centers and 32.5% of community health centers did so.

3.6 Capacity for intervention and management of the NCDs prevention and control

3.6.1 Major NCDs and risk factor intervention

In 2011, the proportion of the CDCs at each level implementng or participating in personalized intervention for high risk population exposed to NCDs、rose to 28.1%, compared with 2009 (13.7%). Specifically, 64.1% for hypertension, 62.8% for diabetes, 21.4% for malignant tumor, 15.1% for stroke, 14.3% for coronary heart disease, and 8.7% for COPD (chronic obstructive pulmonary disease), all witnessed an increase compared with 2009 (the proportion was respectively 36.1%, 32.2%, 16.1%, 10.9%, 11.0% and 6.5%).

In 2011, nationwide, 35.2%, 24.7%, 20.7% and 16.2% of the CDCs, respectively implemented intervention targeting at intervention programs or work related to tobacco use, diet, physical activity, and alcohol use, which saw an obvious growth compared with 2009 (the proportion was respectively 18.4%, 15.4%, 12.2%, and 9.3%).

The same year, 20.2%, 33.4%, 31.8% and 16.2% of the CDCs respectively implemented intervention targeting at overweight and obesity, hypertension, raised blood glucose, and dyslipidemia, an obvious rise tendency compared with 2009 (the proportion is respectively 11.5%, 19.9%, 17.2% and 9.9%).

3.6.2 Early detection for chronic disease patients and high risk populations

In 2011, 94.1% of PHCUs conducted screening of hypertension among patients aged 35 and above during their first visit to a health care institution for medical purposes, among which 89. 1% of the community health centers and 94. 1% of the town public health centers did so, which experienced an obvious rising stage compared with 2009 (such proportions in 2009 were respectively 89. 1% and 43. 8%).

In 2011, 93. 4% of the community health centers and 90. 9% of the town public health centers provided free medical examination for the elderly aged 65 and above, which faced an obvious increase compared with 2009 (74. 8% and 45. 0% respectively). The free examinations varied as follows: 99. 9% of the institutions measured blood pressure, 98. 8% measured weight, 98. 7% measured height, 95. 5% measured blood glucose, 93. 0% measured waist circumference, 80. 9% implemented electrocardiography measurement, and 64. 9% measured blood fat and 36. 6% conduct X-ray examination.

3. 6. 3 Management of patients suffering from and high risk populations exposed to major NCDs

In 2011, 96. 8% of the surveyed PHCUs established health records for hypertension patients, which was apparently higher than 2009 (62. 8%). 44. 0% of the surveyed institutions have set up health records for those whose blood pressure was normal apparently higher than 2009 (26. 8%). Among the surveyed institutions, 96. 0% have implemented follow-up management for hypertensive and 34. 3% have carried out follow-up management of people with normal blood pressure. As estimated, the management rate for hypertension patients was 14. 2%, the standard management rate for managed population was 82. 6% and the control rate was 53. 1% in the jurisdiction where the PHCUs responsible for the hypertension management lie (a growth tendency compared with 2009: 12. 0%, 73. 8% and 48. 7%).

In 2011, 95. 6% of the surveyed PHCUs carried out the establishment of health records for diabetes and 28. 2% of the institutions have set up health records for people who exposed to high diabetes risk, such as people with impaired fasting blood glucose or impaired glucose tolerance. These two proportions both increased compared with 2009 (respectively 61. 3% and 15. 5%). Among the said institutions, 94. 7% have implemented follow-up management for diabetes and 15. 5% do so for people with impaired fasting blood glucose or impaired glucose tolerance. As estimated, PHCUs carrying out diabetes management, the management rate of diabetes was 10. 1%, the rate of standard management of managed populations was 82. 5% and the control rate was 51. 7% (the proportions were respectively 7. 9%, 80. 1% and 50. 0% in 2009).

3. 6. 4 Capacity to provide rehabilitative services for NCDs

In 2011, among the surveyed PHCUs, 676 (22. 9%) have implemented mechanical rehabilitative services for patients with stroke, while 38. 6% of the community health centers and 7. 1% of the town public health centers did so.

3.7 Capacity to assess NCDs

In 2011, 30.6% CDCs or health administrations have carried out assessment of the responses to the prevention and control of NCDs in their respective jurisdictions, which was remarkably higher than that in 2009 (13.3%). The proportion at the provincial level was 37.5%, a slight decline compared with 2009 (40.6%) but higher than the municipal level (29.8%) and the county/district level (30.6%), both obviously higher than 2009, 19.7% and 12.2%, respectively.

In 2011, nationwide, 71.1% of the whole CDCs get involved in the evaluation or performance assessment applicable for PHCUs in their respective jurisdictions, which proportion was apparently higher than that in 2009 (40.9%). Such proportion at the provincial/municipal/county/district levels was 71.9%, 70.8% and 71.2%, which was higher than that in 2009, 62.5%, 45.1% and 40.2%, respectively.

3.8 Capacity for NCDs research

Nationwide, 6.7% CDCs served as principal investigator or participants of research on the prevention and control of NCDs funded by the national agencies in 2011, slightly higher than 2009 (6.1%). In 2011, nationwide, only 1.1% CDCs participated in NCDs research funded by international agencies, lower than the findings in 2009 (3.8%). Nationwide, only 8.3% CDCs published articles either in domestic journals or international peer-reviewed journals in 2011, slightly lower than 2009 (9.7%). In 2011, nationwide, only 27 CDCs (0.8%) published monographs on NCDs, lower than 2009 (4.8%). In 2011, 27 CDCs (0.8%) were granted with national scientific and technological advancement award, 12.5% of the CDCs were the provincial level ones, 3.8% at the municipal level, and 0.3% at the county/district level (in comparison with 2009, the corresponding proportions were 12.5%, 5.8% and 2.7%).

3.9 Comprehensive NCDs capacity

If we draw core indicators from the previously assessed eight modules, we can summarize as follows: ①Three indicators on the policy capacity module, including Indicator 1 (information on the deployment of special fiscal funds appropriated by the Government for the prevention and control of NCDs), Indicator 2 (information on proposals or bills with the subject of the prevention and control of NCDs) and Indicator 3 {information on the formulation (by the Government or multiple departments) of comprehensive plan on the prevention and control of NCDs}; ②Three indicators on basic deployment capacity module, including Indicator 4 (information on the setting of the special division on the prevention and control of NCDs), Indicator 5 (information on the proportion of full-time personnel in health technical personnel responsible for disease control engaged in the prevention and control of NCDs) and Indicator 6 (information on the equipment of glucose meters and sphygmomanometers); ③ Three indicators on education, training and direction capacity, including Indicator 7 (information on the holding of workshops related to the prevention and control of NCDs), Indicator 8 (information on the direction by CDCs of the county level over PHCUs) and Indicator 9 (information on the holding of health lectures by PHCUs); ④Two cooperation modules, including Indicator 10 (information on the cooperation between disease control institutions and media) and Indicator 11 (information on multi-department cooperation); ⑤Three indicators on the early detection and surveillance, including Indicator 12 (information on conducting death cause surveillance across all populations), Indicator 13 (information on conducting risk factor surveillance) and Indicator 14 (information on PHCUs conducting screening of hypertension among patients aged 35 and above during their first visit to a health care institution for medical purposes); ⑥Four intervention and management capacity modules, including Indicator 15 (information on conducting actions on all nationals practicing a healthy life style), Indicator 16 (information on control by PHCUs of hypertension patients' blood pressure), Indicator 17 (information on control by PHCUs of diabetes' blood glucose level) and Indicator 18 (information on two-way referral of hypertension patients and diabetes simultaneously conducted by PHCUs); ⑦ One appraisal capacity module, Indicator 19 (information on the prevention and control of NCDs being taken into consideration when examining or appraising basic medical health service units); One scientific research capacity module, Indicator 20 (information on publishing essays by personnel engaged in the prevention and control of NCDs per capita). The above 20 core indicators make up the comprehensive appraisal indicator system on capacity for the prevention and control of NCDs, with each indicator assigned 5 points, 100 points in total. Each province/autonomous region/municipality directly under the central government, Xinjiang Production and Construction Corps will be graded and sorted in respect of their comprehensive capacity for the prevention and control of NCDs according to their performance of each indicator.

4. Main findings

4.1 Compared with the survey results carried out in 2009, the 2011 survey results indicated that national capacity on policies for NCDs prevention and control, though still weak, has improved. More emphasis remains to be laid on NCDs prevention and control by governments of each level. The prevention and control of NCDs in each locality lacks strong policy guarantee.

4.2 Compared with 2009, the proportion of special divisions responsible for NCDs prevention and control set up at the municipal/county/district level has increased. There were altogether 9315 people working for the prevention and control of NCDs nationwide, 1052 and 1832 more people than 2009 and 2008 respectively, while the proportion of the whole personnel engaged in NCDs prevention and control also took on the tendency of increase (4.2% in 2009 and 4.0% in 2008, respectively). In 2011, the quality of the team engaged in NCDs prevention and control has further improved, personnel engaged in NCDs prevention and control with a bachelor's degree or above accounting for 43. 7% (in comparison with 38. 2% in 2009 and 34. 7% in 2008, respectively). In 2011, 57. 3% CDCs nationwide were appropriated with funds for personnel engaged in NCDs prevention and control, with a certain increase compared with 2009 (40. 2%), though the amount of deployment differs remarkably among the CDCs of different levels and regions and funds for personnel engaged in NCDs prevention and control only accounted for 4. 4% of the disease control funds, which saw an increase compared with that in 2009 (2. 7%). In 2011, among the surveyed basic medical health service units, there was a large increase in terms of the rate of each kind of equipment on NCDs prevention and control at town public health centers compared with 2009, whereas this rate remains below that at community health centers in addition to X-ray machines.

4. 3 Nationwide, 67. 2% of the CDCs of each level hold training on NCDs prevention and control in 2011, 23. 7% higher than 2009 (43. 5%). In 2011, people from each-level CDCs nationwide attending training on NCDs prevention and control reached 78. 5%, 24. 7% higher than 2009 (53. 8%). In 2011, each-level CDCs had high demand for expertise training. Only by providing targeted training according to specific demand of CDCs of each level can such training achieve far better effect. As for the proportion of which holds related activities, town public health centers fell behind community health centers, and in respect of the capacity for knowledge popularity, town public health centers were lower than community health centers.

4. 4 In 2011, the degree of cooperation between CDCs of each level and other departments was higher than that in 2009, but the proportion remained at a low level, especially between CDCs of the county/district level and other institutions. In 2011, in NCDs prevention and control, main cooperation institutions were still mass media and level 2 or above hospitals, the degree of which was apparently higher than other institutions. The rate of cooperation between CDCs of each level and each type of institutions engaged in NCDs prevention and control took on a declining tendency in 2011 both on the part of the province/municipal/county/district level and on the part of the eastern, middle and western districts in China, which essentially consistent with the one in 2009.

4. 5 The surveillance of various NCDs was carried out at a lower proportion on the whole. The surveillance level especially at the basic institutions requires improving. The relevant surveillance of NCDs prevention and control house already been conducted, the proportion of which covering all counties/districts/streets/towns was above 50% and the one can better reflect on the real situation in the monitored region, is typical of local representativeness. In 2011, in the relevant surveillance of all kinds of NCDs already conducted, compilation of annual reports remains the main form of information dissemination and use.

4. 6 Compared with 2009, a higher proportion of CDCs of each level were engaged in NCDs

prevention and control and intervention in risk factors in 2011, although the overall level remained low. The systems on screening of hypertension among patients aged 35 and above during their first visit to a health care institution for medical purposes and on free medical examination for the elderly aged 65 and above have been preliminarily in place in PHCUs. The capacity of town public health centers for early detection has remarkably improved compared with 2009. The proportion of PHCUs that assumed the management of hypertension patients and diabetics was by far higher than that in 2009. Although the management rate in jurisdictions was higher, the efforts are dwarfed by immense crowds of patients and standard management process and management effect remained to be improved. The management of people at high risk has improved to a certain degree compared with 2009 although which was still low.

4.7 In 2011, the CDCs or health administrations of the municipal and county/district levels became strengthened compared with 2009 in terms of their capacity evaluation for coping with NCDs prevention and control. A higher proportion of CDCs of each level, which was over 70%, a remarkable growth compared with 2009, participate in the examination and appraisal by PHCUs. Such proportion saw an upward trend at different extents on the part of the provincial/municipal/county/district levels respectively.

4.8 Provincial CDCs are typical of stronger scientific research capacity for NCDs prevention and control, apparently stronger than those at the municipal/county/district level. The scientific research capacity for NCDs prevention and control in the eastern region is stronger than that in the middle and western parts of China. However, the scientific capacity for NCDs prevention and control, nationwide, remains weak.

5. Policy Suggestions

5.1 Strengthening policy advocacy and equalizing regional development.

5.2 Steadily improving basic deployment for NCDs prevention and control.

5.3 Improving the work ability of NCDs prevention and control at the basic level by taking advantage of the advantages on provincial technical training and direction capability.

5.4 Intensifying cross-departmental cooperation and improving the capacity for decision making related to NCDs prevention and control.

5.5 Doing a good job in basic work for NCDs prevention and control to ensure work quality.

5.6 Improving the capacity evaluation each-level CDCs for coping with NCDs prevention and control and actively carrying out scientific cooperation.

目　录

第一章 绪 论

一、调查背景

目前，以恶性肿瘤、心脑血管疾病、慢性呼吸系统疾病和糖尿病为代表的慢性病已经成为我国居民的主要死因。全国第三次死因调查显示，我国前四位的死因为脑血管病、恶性肿瘤、呼吸系统疾病和心脏病，慢性病死亡率为503/10万。1973~2009年，慢性病占中国人群死因构成由53%上升到85%。与此同时，慢性病还给我国社会造成巨大的经济负担，2005年慢性病医疗费用为14 762亿元人民币，慢性病占疾病负担比例由1993年的54%上升至2005年的63%。由于慢性病为终身性疾病，巨大的直接经济成本和劳动力丧失导致的间接经济成本必将给个人、家庭和整个社会带来沉重的负担，影响社会经济的健康发展。因此，从国家层面采取有力措施加大对慢性病的控制力度，减少疾病危害，降低疾病经济负担，十分必要。

对慢性病预防控制能力进行的调查将能在一定程度上反映我国慢性病防控工作的基本情况和现有的应对能力，发现目前慢性病防控工作中的不足，进而确定今后工作的重点和加强慢性病防控能力建设，为更好地预防和控制慢性病服务。2001年和2005年世界卫生组织（WHO）在191个成员国中开展了两次全球慢性病预防控制能力调查。2001年和2006年东南亚地区组织了两次东南亚地区各国慢性病预防控制能力调查。美洲地区也在地区慢性病预防控制能力评估方面做了相应的工作，并提出了慢性病防控能力应该考虑的七个主题：策略、合作、信息、教育、新颖、交流和评估。在国家层面，加拿大在2004年10月~2005年4月期间组织了一次慢性病预防控制组织能力调查，这是第一个在国家范围内开展的公共卫生系统慢性病预防控制组织能力调查。2009年4月，WHO在总结以往慢性病防控能力调查工作的基础上公布了最新的慢性病预防控制能力评估框架，主要包括以下六个模块：第一，公共卫生系统内慢性病防控的基础设施（包括慢性病防控机构设置、人力资源配置、慢性病防控经费来源和配置）；第二，慢性病相关的政策、策略、行动计划、规划；第三，卫生信息系统、慢性病的监测和调查；第四，针对慢性病社会决定因素的健康促进行动方案；第五，医疗卫生系统慢性病早期发现、治疗、康复的能力；第六，合作情况。综上可见，有越来越多的国际组织、地区和国家重视对慢性病预防控制能力的评估工作。

在我国，防控慢性病的技术工作主要由各级疾控中心和基层医疗卫生机构承担，这些机构防控慢性病的能力直接关系到我国慢性病预防控制工作的成效，但长期以来我们对这些机构的基础设施、人员配置、经费配置和开展工作的现状缺乏全面系统的了解。2009 年 2 月~5 月，中国疾控中心以全国 31 个省（自治区、直辖市）的省级、地市级和县（区）级疾控中心为调查对象开展了一次全国疾控系统慢性病防控基本情况调查，基本摸清了我国各级疾控中心慢性病防控的机构、人力资源、能力培训、开展的工作、经费、合作等情况。在总结 2009 年调查结果的基础上，中国疾控中心设立专门的工作团队，查阅相关文献，结合我国实际情况，根据慢性病防控策略和我国慢性病防控工作重点和工作体系特点，制定和发展了慢性病防控能力评估框架，初步建立了我国慢性病防控能力评估指标体系，并应用这些指标设计了 2010 年全国慢性病预防控制能力调查问卷，利用网络填报的方式，组织开展了 2010 年全国慢性病防控能力调查，收集了 2009 年全国各级疾控中心和 1200 家基层医疗卫生机构慢性病防控能力数据。

2011 年是我国深化医药卫生体制改革中“2009~2011 年着力抓好五项重点改革”工作的最后一年，也是反映“医改”工作阶段性成效的关键一年。在总结 2010 年全国慢性病防控能力调查工作经验的基础上，中国疾控中心继续沿用 2010 年全国慢性病防控能力调查问卷基本框架，调整部分调查内容，进一步完善能力调查网报系统，组织开展 2012 年全国慢性病防控能力调查，主要收集调查对象 2011 年慢性病防控能力情况。

本次调查旨在能更加全面地反映目前我国慢性病防控能力现状，为进一步加强国家慢性病防控能力建设、构建更加完善的慢性病防控体系提供可靠的依据。

二、调查目的

系统评估 2011 年我国慢性病防控能力现状及慢性病防控能力建设中的制约因素和需求情况；并与 2009 年调查结果作对比，了解我国慢性病防控能力变化情况；综合评估各省慢性病防控能力；为落实国家基本公共卫生服务项目提供基线数据，为加强我国慢性病防控能力建设、制定慢性病防控相关政策提供依据。

三、调查内容与方法

（一）慢性病防控相关政策能力调查

1. 调查对象

全国 31 个省、自治区、直辖市及新疆生产建设兵团各级卫生行政部门和疾控中心从事慢性病防控工作的关键人员，包括各级卫生厅（局）疾控处（科）分管慢病的领导、疾控中心分管慢病的主任和承担慢病防控工作的科所长。

2. 调查内容

主要包括以下几个方面：

（1）当地政策问题认识能力

政府或卫生行政部门慢性病防控专项财政经费、政府领导参加慢性病防控活动情况、两会上以慢性病防控为主题的提案或议案等。

（2）当地政策制定能力

政府或卫生行政部门制定或转发的现行慢性病防控相关规划、工作（实施）方案、规范或指南的情况。

3. 调查组织形式

各省、地市、区（县），由卫生厅（局）疾控处（科）分管慢病的领导、疾控中心分管慢病的主任和承担慢病防控工作的科所长 3 人组成调查小组，具体调查工作由科所长负责联系。如果各地市或区（县）级疾控中心没有具体承担慢病防控工作的科所，则由中心办公室的主任/副主任负责联系。

（二）疾控机构慢性病防控能力调查

1. 调查对象

全国 31 个省、自治区、直辖市及新疆生产建设兵团各级卫生行政部门和疾控中心从事慢性病防控工作的关键人员，包括各级卫生厅（局）疾控处（科）分管慢病的领导、疾控中心分管慢病的主任和承担慢病防控工作的科所长。

2. 调查内容

主要包括以下几个方面：

（1）基本情况。

（2）机构基础配置能力

部门设置：承担慢性病防控工作的主要部门的性质；除承担慢性病防控工作的主要部门外，承担慢性病防控工作的业务部门数量。

人力资源配置：慢性病防控（专职）人员的数量、所占比例、工作经验、学历、技术职称、执业资格等。

经费配置：慢性病业务工作经费的数额及占总业务经费的比例；各种来源的慢性病防控经费数额及所占比例。

（3）机构参与能力

参与本级卫生行政部门慢性病防控政策制定的情况；参与本级政府或其他行政部门（卫生行政部门除外）慢性病防控相关工作（政策制定、会议、活动）的情况；参与上级卫生行政部门或上级疾控中心慢性病防控相关政策制定的情况。

（4）机构教育培训与指导能力

举办培训：主办各级培训班的次数、培训人次数；其中举办继续教育培训的次数和培训人次数。

接受进修：接受外单位进修的人次数。

参加培训：参加培训的次数、人次数；其中参加继续教育培训的次数和人次数。

培训需求：慢性病防控培训需求情况（统计分析、死因监测、慢性病及危险因素监测技能培训、慢性病干预管理技能培训、慢性病防控基础及综合培训）。

现场工作（技术）指导：省、地市疾控中心对县（区）级疾控中心开展现场指导的次数，指导的机构数；县（区）级疾控中心对基层医疗卫生机构开展现场指导的次数，指导的机构数。

（5）机构合作能力

卫生领域内，本地区开展慢性病防控工作的单位（CDC、独立的健康教育所、医院、基层医疗卫生机构、专业防治机构、NGO、社会团体等）。

卫生领域外，本地区参与慢性病防控工作的部门（体育、教育、发改、财政、人社、农业、工信、计生、环境、广电等）。

本单位与媒体、医院、专业防办、大学院校、科研院所、企业、NGO 等机构（部门）的合作情况。

（6）监测能力

慢性病相关监测/登记工作（死因监测、恶性肿瘤病例报告、脑卒中病例报告、心肌梗死病例报告）的开展情况：当地是否开展、被调查单位是否承担、工作任务来源、覆盖县区数、覆盖街道/乡镇数、是否有当地代表性、资料收集途径、数据更新情况、数据发布及利用、信息采纳情况、是否评估、评估后是否调整。

慢性病危险因素相关监测包含的指标（吸烟、膳食、身体活动、饮酒、超重和肥胖、血压、血糖和血脂）情况：当地是否开展、被调查单位是否承担、工作任务来源、覆盖区县数、覆盖街道/乡镇数、是否有当地代表性、数据获取方式、开展频次、数据发布及利用、信息采纳情况、是否评估、评估后是否调整。

根据现有监测、调查系统获得当地代表性指标的情况。

（7）干预能力

慢性病患者（高血压、糖尿病、恶心肿瘤、脑卒中、冠心病、慢性呼吸系统疾病）或高危人群的个体化干预情况：是否开展、任务来源、承担角色、干预环节、干预场所、工作频次、干预方案的评估及评估后的调整。

慢性病危险因素人群干预（全民健康生活方式行动、烟草使用、膳食、身体活动、酒精使用、超重或肥胖、血压升高、血糖升高、血脂异常）情况：是否开展、任务来源、针对人群、干预手段、干预场所、工作频次、干预方案的评估及评估后的调整。

（8）评估能力

是否开展评估、是否形成评估报告、评估报告的内容、评估报告发放范围、是否参与基层医疗卫生机构考核（评估）等。

（9）科研能力

包括科研课题、发表论文、出版专著、科技成果等情况。

3. 调查组织形式

各省、地市、区县，由卫生厅（局）疾控处（科）分管慢性病的领导、疾控中心分管慢性病的主任和承担慢病防控工作的科所长 3 人组成调查小组，具体调查工作由科所长负责联系。如果各地市和区县级疾控中心没有具体承担慢病防控工作的科所，则由中心办公室的主任/副主任负责联系。

（三）基层医疗卫生机构慢性病防控能力抽样调查

1. 调查对象

被抽中的基层医疗卫生机构的负责人和有关科室负责人。

2. 抽样方法

根据《2011 年中国卫生统计年鉴》显示全国共有 6903 家社区卫生服务中心和 37 836 家乡镇卫生院。本次调查利用中国疾病预防控制信息系统中基层医疗卫生机构的数据进行完全随机抽样，分别抽取 1500 家社区卫生服务中心和 1500 家乡镇卫生院作为调查对象。

3. 调查内容

主要包括以下几个方面：

（1）基本情况

（2）基础配置

设备配置能力、人力资源能力、经费配置能力。

（3）培训、指导情况

举办、参加培训的情况；开展现场技术指导的情况；存有各级现行慢性病防控相关规范或指南的情况。

培训需求：开展慢性病防控工作培训需求情况（诊疗技能培训、患者管理技能培训、健康教育技能培训、数据利用培训、报病技能培训等）。

（4）参与慢性病防控相关项目或科研工作的情况。

（5）慢性病防控知识普及情况

主要慢性病健康日期间开展相关宣传活动的情况；举办健康教育知识讲座的情况；制作宣传册的情况。

（6）慢性病患者及高危人群早期发现

开展 35 岁以上居民首诊测血压、45 岁以上居民免费血糖检测、65 岁以上老年人免费健康体检工作的情况。

（7）主要慢性病病例报告

开展新发脑卒中病例报告、急性心肌梗死病例报告、死亡病例报告的情况。

（8）患者和高危人群登记、随访管理

开展高血压（糖尿病）患者、高危人群建档和随访管理工作的情况；高血压（糖尿病）患者自我管理小组建立情况；居民委员会、村民委员会参与高血压（糖尿病）患者随访管理工作的情况；高血压（糖尿病）患者转诊情况。

4. 调查组织形式

由各县区级疾控中心承担慢性病防控工作的科所长走访本县区内被抽中的基层医疗卫生机构，询问基层医疗卫生机构的负责人和有关科室负责人。县区级疾控中心慢病分管主任确保联系畅通。

四、数据采集方式

本次调查继续采用网络调查的形式，中国疾控中心信息采集平台上搭建了2012年全国慢性病防控能力调查网络填报系统。系统包括2012年全国慢性病防控能力调查疾控系统调查表和2012年全国慢性病防控能力调查基层医疗卫生机构调查表。各级疾控中心通过用户名和密码登录平台，填写本单位调查表，县（区）级疾控中心同时负责填写基层医疗卫生机构调查表。

五、职责分工

（一）中国疾控中心

全面负责调查工作：

1. 设计调查方案和调查问卷。
2. 完善在线能力调查系统。
3. 负责组织培训省级调查协调员。
4. 负责组织现场督导工作。
5. 负责收集、汇总各省录入完毕的调查数据。
6. 分析调查数据、撰写调查报告。

（二）省级疾控中心

省级疾控中心慢性病防控科所负责具体联系组织本省调查工作：

1. 负责协调本级调查小组成员参与调查，并指定专人负责填写本级调查表和完成在线录入填报。

2. 负责组织本省各级调查工作。

3. 指定专门人员（经国家疾控中心培训的调查协调员）作为咨询员解答本省各级在调查表填写过程中的疑问，必要时开展相关培训。

4. 负责收集本省各级盖章的诚信说明，并对本省的调查表进行在线审核和抽查。

5. 必要时，配合中国疾控中心对省内的部分地区开展现场督导。

（三）地市级疾控中心

地市级疾控中心承担慢性病防控工作的科所（没有该类科所的中心由中心办公室负责）具体联系组织做好本市调查工作：

1. 负责组织本级调查小组成员填写本级调查表，完成在线录入填报。

2. 确认完成在线调查后，将本地市纸质调查表封面盖章后邮寄至本省疾控中心。

3. 配合省级疾控中心协调做好本地市各县（区）疾控中心的调查工作。

4. 必要时，配合上级对地市内的部分县区开展现场督导。

（四）县（区）级疾控中心

县（区）级疾控中心承担慢性病防控工作的科所（没有该类科所的中心由中心办公室负责）具体联系组织做好本县（区）调查工作：

1. 负责组织本级调查小组成员填写本级调查表并完成在线录入填报。

2. 承担对本辖区内抽到的社区卫生服务中心和乡镇卫生院进行调查并完成在线录入填报。

3. 确认完成在线调查后，将本县（区）纸质调查表封面盖章后邮寄至本省疾控中心。

4. 必要时，配合上级对县（区）内的部分调查单位开展现场督导。

（五）社区卫生服务中心和乡镇卫生院

1. 配合县（区）级疾控中心开展针对本单位的问卷调查。

2. 必要时，配合各级疾控中心开展现场督导。

六、质量控制

（一）调查前

1. 调查方案论证

组织专家对调整后的调查方案和调查表进行论证，保证调查的科学性及可行性。

2. 系统填报测试。

3. 培训

组织对省级疾控中心的调查协调员进行培训，调查协调员要作为咨询员解答本省各级在调查表填写过程中的疑问，确保调查数据的质量。

（二）调查过程中

1. 调查员和审核员

各级疾控中心指定2~3名熟悉本级慢性病防控工作的人员组成调查小组：填表员负责填写问卷；审核员负责对填表员填写好的调查表进行审核，发现问题及时更改、补充，保证填写内容符合本单位实际情况。

2. 被调查单位

作为调查对象的社区卫生服务中心和乡镇卫生院，其被访人员要由熟悉本单位慢性病防控工作的多名工作人员组成，成员必须包括机构的负责人，配合县级疾控中心完成对本单位的调查。

3. 督导

在中国疾病中心的统一协调下，开展逐级、跨级督导工作，以确保调查的质量。

4. 复核

省级疾控中心慢性病防控科所对本省数据进行审核，并抽取本省5%的调查对象［包括地市和县（区）级疾控中心、社区卫生服务中心和乡镇卫生院］，对其调查表的填写内容进行检查，对与常理或实际情况不符的内容及时反馈，并由原填写人员核实，修改或解释。

（三）数据处理过程中

1. 数据库建立

由中国疾控中心编制在线录入填报系统。

2. 数据录入

由各级疾控中心负责在线数据录入，省级疾控中心负责审核和抽查。

七、数据清理与分析方法

（一）数据清理

依据数据清理方案编写标准程序进行数据库清理，产生清理后用于分析的数据库。针对记录，清理重复记录；针对变量，根据各个变量的值域及意义对错误值（缺失、逻辑错误、异常）进行清理，对所有含有缺失值、逻辑错误和异常值的变量进行标记，原则上不删除任何记录，在对相应变量进行分析时，不包括这些记录。

（二）分析方法

用SAS和SPSS统计软件分别对各部分进行分析，主要采用描述性分析方法。

第二章　分析结果

一、数据完成情况

本次调查全国3340家疾控中心，包括省级32家，地市级347家，县（区）级2961家和3000家基层医疗卫生机构（包括1500家社区卫生服务中心和1500家乡镇卫生院）。在线调查结束时，共有32家省级疾控中心、346家地市级疾控中心、2937家县（区）级疾控中心和2955家基层医疗卫生机构填写了完整的调查问卷，应答率分别为100%、99.7%、99.2%和98.5%（表2-1、表2-2、表2-3）。本次被调查疾控机构总应答率为99.3%，高于2009年（97.2%），基层医疗卫生机构的应答率也高于2009（96.4%）。

表2-1　全国各级疾控中心应答情况

级别	机构数	应答数	应答率（%）
省级	32	32	100
地市级	347	346	99.7
县（区）级	2961	2937	99.2
合计	**3340**	**3315**	**99.3**

表2-2　全国各省疾控中心应答情况

省（自治区、直辖市）	机构数	应答数	应答率（%）
北京	19	19	100
天津	19	19	100
河北	188	188	100
山西	131	131	100
内蒙古	113	112	99.1
辽宁	120	120	100
吉林	66	66	100
黑龙江	146	146	100
上海	19	19	100

续 表

省（自治区、直辖市）	机构数	应答数	应答率（%）
江苏	125	125	100
浙江	100	100	100
安徽	117	115	98.3
福建	96	96	100
江西	111	111	100
山东	159	159	100
河南	181	181	100
湖北	101	101	100
湖南	145	144	99.3
广东	126	125	99.2
广西	103	101	98.1
海南	23	23	100
重庆	39	39	100
四川	205	205	100
贵州	99	99	100
云南	146	146	100
西藏	82	73	89.0
陕西	119	119	100
甘肃	102	99	97.1
青海	55	49	89.1
宁夏	25	25	100
新疆	109	109	100
新疆建设兵团	151	151	100
合计	**3340**	**3315**	**99.3**

表 2-3 全国各省基层医疗卫生机构应答情况

省（自治区、直辖市）	机构数	应答数	应答率（%）
北京	85	85	100
天津	69	69	100
河北	104	104	100
山西	84	84	100

续　表

省（自治区、直辖市）	机构数	应答数	应答率（%）
内蒙古	96	95	99.0
辽宁	107	107	100
吉林	71	71	100
黑龙江	83	82	98.8
上海	72	72	100
江苏	215	214	99.5
浙江	166	165	99.4
安徽	131	126	96.2
福建	91	91	100
江西	78	78	100
山东	107	106	99.1
河南	123	123	100
湖北	105	105	100
湖南	133	129	97.0
广东	116	114	98.3
广西	68	62	91.2
海南	16	16	100
重庆	87	87	100
四川	273	273	100
贵州	100	100	100
云南	81	81	100
西藏	29	28	96.6
陕西	112	108	96.4
甘肃	112	94	84.0
青海	16	16	100
宁夏	14	14	100
新疆	50	50	100
新疆建设兵团	6	6	100
合计	3000	2955	98.5

二、慢性病防控政策能力

慢性病防控政策主要指慢性病防控相关规划、方案等政策性文件。慢性病防控政策能力主要包括慢性病防控政策认定能力、政策制定能力、政策执行能力、政策评估能力和政策调整能力等。考虑到数据的可获得性和实际意义等因素，只针对各地、各级慢性病防控政策认定能力和制定能力进行分析和评价。

（一）政策认定能力

政策认定能力，即将社会问题转化为政策问题的能力。本调查中主要包括政府经费支持（各级慢性病防控专项财政经费数额）、政府领导参与（各级政府领导参与慢性病防控相关活动数量）和政策倡导（各级两会慢性病防控相关提案或议案的数量）三方面。

1. 财政经费支持情况

财政经费支持情况主要指被调查单位所在地区本级政府或卫生行政部门财政预算中配置慢性病防控专项经费的情况。

2011 年，全国省级财政经费中配置慢性病防控专项经费的比例为 84.4%，地市级和县（区）级分别为 28.0%和 21.5%；省级经费配置比例明显高于地市级和县（区）级。配置专项经费的比例均呈现东部（34.1%）、中部（19.0%）、西部（17.1%）递减的趋势，各级疾控中心均是如此（表 2-4）。

与 2009 年调查结果比较，各级经费配置比例均有所上升（2009 年省市县三级依次为 75%、19.7%和 11.3%）。

表 2-4 各地、各级财政预算中配置有慢性病防控专项经费的情况 [机构数（%）]

级别	东部	中部	西部	合计
省级	10（90.9）	7（87.5）	10（76.9）	27（84.4）
地市级	49（50.0）	21（20.2）	27（18.8）	97（28.0）
县（区）级	280（31.7）	161（18.2）	190（16.2）	631（21.5）
合计	**339（34.1）**	**189（19.0）**	**227（17.1）**	**755（22.8）**

各级财政慢性病防控专项经费的数额，省级平均为 311.4 万元（2009 年为 113.9 万元），地市级平均为 104.0 万元（2009 年为 27.3 万元），县（区）级平均为 80.9 万元（2009 年为 41.8 万元），三级政府投入的经费均有较大程度增加（表 2-5）。从地区分布来看，东部地区专项经费的均值和中位数均高于中、西部地区，西部地区均值高于中部地区（表 2-6）。

表 2-5 各级财政预算中慢性病防控专项经费情况（万元，人民币）

级别	最大值	最小值	平均数	中位数
省级	2900.0	5.0	311.4	135.0
地市级	4200.0	0.4	104.0	10.0
县（区）级	3929.8	0.1	80.9	13.8

表 2-6 各地财政预算中慢性病防控专项经费的情况（万元，人民币）

地区	最大值	最小值	平均值	中位数
东部	3929.8	0.1	132.2	20.0
中部	800.0	0.2	43.7	10.0
西部	4200.0	0.1	72.7	10.0
合计	**4200.0**	**0.1**	**92.1**	**14.0**

2. 政府领导参与情况

以各级政府领导参与慢性病防控相关活动的情况为衡量，主要包括慢性病防控相关新闻发布会、慢性病防控相关现场活动和慢性病防控相关工作会议等。

省、地市、县（区）级政府领导参与慢性病防控相关活动的比例分别为 46.9%、40.8%和 36.1%，除省级较 2009 年有所降低外，地市和县（区）级均有所增加［2009 年省、地市、县（区）三级分别为 53.1%、29.8%和 20.8%］。省级疾控中心中部地区领导参与比例最高，地市级疾控中心东部地区领导参与比例最高，县（区）级疾控中心西部地区领导参与比例最低，见表 2-7。就具体参与活动的类型来看，政府领导参加慢性病相关新闻发布会、现场活动和工作会议的比例分别为 8.1%、83.2%和 73.2%（表 2-8、表 2-9、表 2-10）。

表 2-7 各地、各级政府有领导参加各类慢性病防控相关活动的情况［数量（%）］

级别	东部	中部	西部	合计
省级	5（45.5）	5（62.5）	5（38.5）	15（46.9）
地市级	52（53.1）	47（45.2）	42（29.2）	141（40.8）
县（区）级	348（39.4）	350（39.6）	362（30.9）	1060（36.1）

政府领导参加新闻发布会比例较低，且省、地市和县（区）三级逐级降低（分别为 20%、12.1%和 7.5%），但就参加次数来看，三级差距不大（表 2-8）。

表 2-8 各地、各级政府领导参加慢性病相关新闻发布会的情况

级别	东部		中部		西部		合计	
	机构数（%）	平均数	机构数（%）	平均数	机构数（%）	平均数	机构数（%）	平均数
省级	1（20.0）	1.0	1（20.0）	3.0	1（20.0）	1.0	3（20.0）	1.7
地市级	6（11.5）	1.5	6（12.8）	1.5	5（11.9）	2.8	17（12.1）	1.9
县（区）级	26（7.5）	1.4	34（9.7）	1.9	19（5.2）	1.9	79（7.5）	1.7

省、地市和县（区）三级政府领导参与慢性病相关现场活动呈逐级下降，分别为 93.3%、90.8%和 82.1%，平均参加次数为 2.2 次，三级次数差别不大。中、西部省级政府领导参与现场活动比例均达到 100%，中部地区省级政府领导参与现场活动平均次数达到 3.6 次，明显高于其他地区和市、县两级（表 2-9）。

表 2-9 各地、各级政府领导参加慢性病相关现场活动的情况

级别	东部		中部		西部		合计	
	机构数（%）	平均数	机构数（%）	平均数	机构数（%）	平均数	机构数（%）	平均数
省级	4（80.0）	1.5	5（100.0）	3.6	5（100.0）	1.8	14（93.3）	2.4
地市级	47（90.4）	1.7	42（89.4）	2.1	39（92.9）	2.4	128（90.8）	2.1
县（区）级	288（82.8）	2.1	287（82.5）	2.2	295（81.5）	2.4	870（82.1）	2.2

省级政府领导参加慢性病相关工作会议比例低于地市和县（区）两级，中部地区县（区）级参与比例最低（表 2-10）。

表 2-10 各地、各级政府领导参加慢性病相关工作会议的情况

级别	东部		中部		西部		合计	
	机构数（%）	平均数	机构数（%）	平均数	机构数（%）	平均数	机构数（%）	平均数
省级	3（60.0）	2.0	4（80.0）	4.3	3（60.0）	1.0	10（66.7）	2.6
地市级	35（67.3）	2.1	38（80.9）	1.9	31（73.8）	2.0	104（73.8）	2.0
县（区）级	258（74.1）	2.2	243（69.4）	2.4	275（76.0）	2.5	776（73.2）	2.4

3. 政策倡导

政策倡导主要指各地区、各级两会上提出以慢性病防控为主题的提案或议案的情况。

2009～2011年，各地、各级两会上有以慢性病防控为主题的提案或议案的比例按省（43.8%）、地市（17.9%）、县（区）（5.9%）依次递减，各级比例与2007～2009年相比，省级有所下降，地市和县（区）级有所上升［2007～2009年省、地市和县（区）三级分别为46.9%、14.7%和3.7%］。地区分布均以东、中、西部依次递减，东部地区远远高于中、西部地区。省级两会提案或议案平均10.0个，地市级平均2.2个，县（区）级平均2.4个，省、县（区）两级较2007～2009年有所增加，地市级有所下降［2007～2009年省、地市和县（区）三级分别为平均3.5个、2.5个和1.6个］（表2-11）。

表2-11　各地、各级两会有以慢性病防控为主题的提案或议案情况

级别	东部		中部		西部		合计	
	机构数（%）	平均数	机构数（%）	平均数	机构数（%）	平均数	机构数（%）	平均数
省级	9（81.8）	14.6	2（25.0）	2.0	3（23.1）	1.7	14（43.8）	10.0
地市级	34（34.7）	2.5	17（16.3）	1.7	11（7.6）	2.0	62（17.9）	2.2
县（区）级	82（9.3）	2.8	44（5.0）	1.3	46（3.9）	2.9	172（5.9）	2.4

（二）政策制定能力

政策制定能力主要以所在地区本级政府或卫生行政部门制定并发布现行慢性病防控相关规划的情况为衡量。慢性病防控相关规划指各级政府或卫生等行政部门（卫生厅局、多部门等）为防控慢性病及其危险因素而制定一段时期的政策性文件，包括慢性病防控综合规划、慢性病防控专病规划和针对慢性病危险因素控制的规划。慢性病防控综合规划指针对至少4类慢性病（心脑血管病、恶性肿瘤、糖尿病和慢性呼吸系统疾病）中的2类，含或不含危险因素（烟草使用、不合理膳食、身体活动不足、酒精使用、超重和肥胖、血压升高、血糖升高、血脂异常）均可。慢性病防控专病规划指专门针对心脑血管疾病、恶性肿瘤、糖尿病和慢性呼吸系统疾病等慢性病中的一类疾病（含或不含危险因素）制定的规划。针对慢性病危险因素控制的规划指专门针对烟草使用、膳食、身体活动、酒精使用、超重或肥胖、血压、血糖、血脂等危险因素中的任何一项或多项的规划。

1. 慢性病防控相关规划

全国共有7个省级（21.9%）、38个地市（11.0%）和432个县（区）（14.7%）颁布了慢性病防控相关规划，省级以西部地区最高（30.8%），地市级和县（区）级均以东部地区最高（分别为12.2%和19.7%）（表2-12）。

表 2-12 各地、各级政府或卫生行政部门有现行慢性病防控相关规划的情况［数量（%）］

级别	东部	中部	西部	合计
省级	2（18.2）	1（12.5）	4（30.8）	7（21.9）
地市级	12（12.2）	11（10.6）	15（10.4）	38（11.0）
县（区）级	174（19.7）	117（13.3）	141（12.1）	432（14.7）
合计	**188（18.9）**	**129（13.0）**	**160（12.1）**	**477（14.4）**

2. 慢性病防控相关工作（实施）方案

2011 年，共有 26 个省级（81.3%）、106 个地市（30.6%）和 753 个县（区）（25.6%）有现行的慢性病防控相关工作（实施）方案。除西部县（区）级有方案的比例高于地市级外，均呈省、地市和县（区）三级和东中西部依次下降趋势（表 2-13）。

表 2-13 各地、各级有现行慢性病防控相关工作（实施）方案的情况［数量（%）］

级别	东部	中部	西部	合计
省级	10（90.9）	7（87.5）	9（69.2）	26（81.3）
地市级	49（50.0）	30（28.8）	27（18.8）	106（30.6）
县（区）级	294（33.3）	203（23.0）	256（21.9）	753（25.6）
合计	**353（35.5）**	**240（24.1）**	**292（22.0）**	**885（26.7）**

三、慢性病防控基础配置能力

慢性病防控基础配置能力主要包括慢性病防控相关部门、人员、经费、设备等的配置情况。

（一）部门设置能力

中国疾控中心于 2002 年成立了慢性非传染性疾病预防控制中心（简称“慢病中心”），并于 2006 年 10 月成立慢性病防治与社区卫生处（简称“慢病社区处”），负责协调中心内多部门联合开展慢性病预防控制工作。2009 年 4 月，控制烟草办公室（简称“控烟办”）独立建制，加强和推进我国履行《烟草控制框架公约》工作。2009 年，中央机构编制委员会办公室批复成立国家癌症中心、国家心血管病中心。至此在全国形成了由中国疾控中心、国家癌症中心、国家心血管病中心、全国脑血管病防治研究办公室、各省及以下各级疾病预防控制中心、专病防治研究办公室、二级以上医院、基层医疗卫生机构组成的慢性病防治网络。

1. 承担慢性病防控工作的部门

2011 年，全国省级和东部地区的地市级疾控中心内均设有承担慢性病防控工作的部门，全国地市级和县区级的设置比例分别为 93. 4%和 89. 2%，较 2009 年有所增加（2009 年该比例分别为 90. 5%和 79. 3%）（表 2-14）。

表 2-14　各地、各级疾控中心设置慢性病防控工作部门的情况［数量（%）］

级别	东部	中部	西部	合计
省级	11（100）	8（100）	13（100）	32（100）
地市级	98（100）	100（96. 2）	125（86. 8）	323（93. 4）
县（区）级	839（94. 9）	835（94. 6）	946（80. 9）	2620（89. 2）
合计	**948（95. 5）**	**943（94. 8）**	**1084（81. 7）**	**2975（89. 7）**

2. 专门的慢性病防控科所

本次调查将承担慢性病防控工作的部门分为 3 类，即专门承担慢性病防控工作的部门、以慢性病防控为主要职责的部门和不以慢性病防控为主要职责的部门。

2011 年，全国省级设立专门慢性病防控科所的比例为 78. 1%，设立以慢性病防控为主要职责的部门的比例为 18. 8%，只有 1 个西部省份设立了承担慢性病防控工作但不作为主要职责的部门（3. 1%），各比例与 2009 年均没有变化。地市级和县（区）级设立专门承担慢性病防控工作的部门的比例明显偏低（分别为 36. 4%和 14. 8%），但较 2009 年有所提高［2009 年地市和县（区）两级比例分别为 27. 2%和 7. 1%］。仍有 46. 3%的县（区）级疾控中心虽然设置了慢性病防控工作部门但其不以慢性病工作为主要职责。从地区分布来看，省、地市和县（区）三级设立专门慢性病防控科所的比例均呈东、中、西部依次下降趋势（表 2-15、表 2-16）。

表 2-15　各级疾控中心设置各类慢性病防控科所［数量（%）］

级别	专门慢性病防控科所	以慢性病防控为主要职责的科所	不以慢性病为主要职责的科所
省级	25（78. 1）	6（18. 8）	1（3. 1）
地市级	126（36. 4）	85（24. 6）	112（32. 4）
县（区）级	436（14. 8）	823（28. 0）	1361（46. 3）

表 2-16 各地疾控中心设置各类慢性病防控科所［数量（%）］

地区	专门慢性病防控科所	以慢性病防控为主要职责的科所	不以慢性病为主要职责的科所
东部	232（23.4）	344（34.6）	372（37.5）
中部	193（19.4）	307（30.9）	443（44.5）
西部	162（12.2）	263（19.8）	659（49.7）
合计	**587（17.7）**	**914（27.6）**	**1474（44.5）**

（二）人力资源能力

人力资源能力包括慢性病防控在岗人员数量、慢性病防控人员年龄、慢性病防控人员工作年限、慢性病防控人员学历、慢性病防控人员所学专业和执业资格等情况。

1. 慢性病防控在岗人员数量

（1）各级疾控中心

慢性病防控在岗人员指 2011 年在岗并承担慢性病防控工作的人员。包括专职人员、承担慢性病防控工作任务的非专职人员，编内和编外人员均计入统计。

截至 2011 年底，全国省、地市和县（区）三级疾控中心慢性病防控在岗人员总人数为 9315 人（占疾控中心总在岗人数的 4.6%），其中省、地市和县（区）三级慢病防控在岗人员分别为 345、1379 和 7591 人，较 2009 年（8263 人，4.2%）和 2008 年（7483 人，4.0%）有所增长（表 2-17 和图 2-1）。

表 2-17 各地、各级疾控中心慢性病防控在岗人员占总体工作人员情况

地区	级别	机构数	疾控中心总在岗人数	慢病防控在岗人员	所占比例（%）
东部	省级	11	5699	175	3.1
	地市级	98	14 381	484	3.4
	县（区）级	884	52 085	2786	5.3
	小计	993	72 165	3445	4.8
中部	省级	8	2732	68	2.5
	地市级	104	13 133	425	3.2
	县（区）级	883	50 592	2302	4.6
	小计	995	66 457	2795	4.2
西部	省级	13	4575	102	2.2
	地市级	144	12 993	470	3.6

续　表

地区	级别	机构数	疾控中心总在岗人数	慢病防控在岗人员	所占比例（%）
	县（区）级	1170	44 860	2503	5.6
	小计	1327	62 428	3075	4.9
合计	省级	32	13 006	345	2.7
	地市级	346	40 507	1379	3.4
	县（区）级	2937	147 537	7591	5.1
	合计	**3315**	**201 050**	**9315**	**4.6**

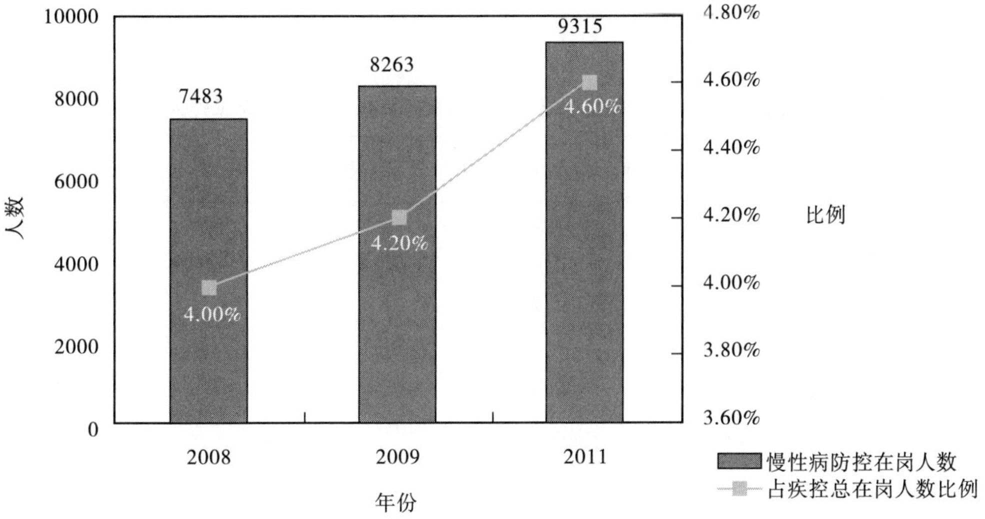

图 2-1　慢性病防控在岗人员数及其占疾控中心总在岗人数比例变化图

全国共 92.3%配置了慢性病防控在岗人员，其中省级配置比例 100%、地市级 96.2%、县（区）级 91.8%，三级平均配置人数分别为 10.8 人、4.1 人和 2.8 人，与 2009 年调查数据相比，省级有所下降，地市级有所上升、县（区）级持平（2009 年三级分别为 11.8 人、3.9 人和 2.8 人）。各级平均慢病防控在岗人数均呈东中西部依次下降（表 2-18）。

表 2-18 各地、各级疾控中心慢性病防控平均在岗人数

级别	东部	中部	西部	合计
省级	15.9	8.5	7.9	10.8
地市级	5	4.1	3.6	4.1
县（区）级	3.2	2.7	2.5	2.8
合计	**3.6**	**2.9**	**2.7**	**3.0**

2011 年，全国省及以下各级疾控中心专职慢性病防控人员总数为 6370 人，省、地市、县（区）三级分别为 310 人、910 人和 4150 人。专职人员占慢病防控在岗人员的 68.4%，占疾控中心总在岗人数的 3.2%，较 2008 年（4796 人，2.6%）和 2009 年（3656 人，1.9%）均有所增加（表 2-19 和图 2-2）。

表 2-19 各地、各级疾控中心专职慢性病防控在岗人员占总在岗工作人员情况

地区	级别	机构数	疾控中心总在岗人数	专职慢病防控在岗人数	所占比例（%）
东部	省级	11	5699	156	2.7
	地市级	98	14 381	350	2.4
	县（区）级	884	52 085	1639	3.1
	小计	993	72 165	2145	3.0
中部	省级	8	2732	64	2.3
	地市级	104	13 133	271	2.1
	县（区）级	883	50 592	1258	2.5
	小计	995	66 457	1593	2.4
西部	省级	13	4575	90	2.0
	地市级	144	12 993	289	2.2
	县（区）级	1170	44 860	1253	2.8
	小计	1327	62 428	1632	2.6
合计	省级	32	13 006	310	2.4
	地市级	346	40 507	910	2.2
	县（区）级	2937	147 537	4150	2.8
	合计	**3315**	**201 050**	**6370**	**3.2**

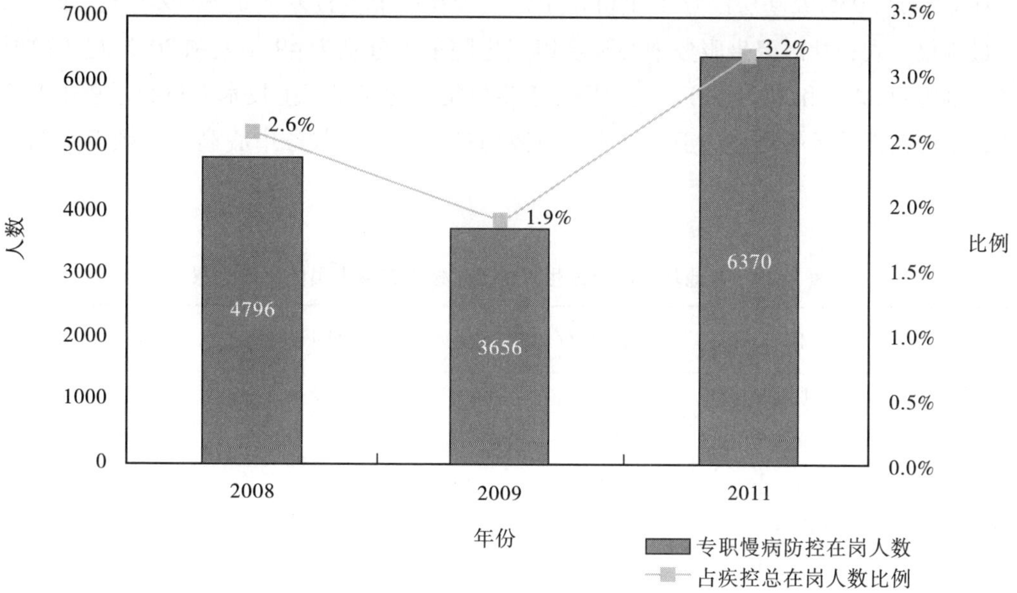

图 2-2 专职慢性病防控在岗人员数及其占疾控中心总在岗人数比例变化图

2011 年，全国省、地市和县（区）三级疾控中心中仅 58%配置了慢病防控专职在岗人员，其中省级配置比例 96.9%、地市级 73.5%、县（区）级 55.8%，三级平均配置人数依次为 10 人、3.6 人和 2.5 人，与 2009 年调查时相比，三级慢病专职在岗人员数均有所上升(2009 年三级分别为 9.5 人、3.2 人和 2.4 人)。各级平均慢病防控专职在岗人数均呈东中西部依次下降（表 2-20）。

表 2-20 各地、各级疾控中心专职慢性病防控平均在岗人数

级别	东部	中部	西部	合计
省级	14	8	7.5	10
地市级	3.9	3.3	3.4	3.6
县（区）级	2.8	2.4	2.4	2.5
合计	3.1	2.6	2.6	2.8

（2）基层医疗卫生机构

基层医疗卫生机构卫生技术在岗人员，包括执业医师、注册护士、药师（士)、检验技师（士)、影响技师（士)、卫生监督员和见习医（药、护、技）师（士）等卫生专业人员，不包括从事管理工作的卫生技术人员（如院长、副院长、党委书记等）。

在应答的 2955 家基层医疗卫生机构中，平均在岗卫生技术人员数 39.8 人，最多 614 人，最少仅 1 人；社区卫生服务中心和乡镇卫生院平均分别为 49.4 人和 30.3 人（2009 年二者分别为 49.2 人和 25.4 人）。基层医疗卫生机构平均在岗卫生技术人员数呈东中西递减趋势；东中西部地区平均在岗卫生技术人员数均是社区卫生服务中心高于乡镇卫生院（表 2-21）。

表 2-21　各地基层医疗卫生机构卫生技术在岗人员的平均数量

地区	类别	应答机构数	最大值	最小值	平均数	中位数
东部	乡镇卫生院	372	614	2	43.4	30
	社区卫生服务中心	771	532	1	60.1	43
	小计	1143	614	1	54.7	39
中部	乡镇卫生院	467	195	2	32.9	26
	社区卫生服务中心	331	264	4	39.3	34
	小计	798	264	2	35.5	29
西部	乡镇卫生院	638	135	1	20.7	15
	社区卫生服务中心	376	291	2	36.3	27
	小计	1014	291	1	26.5	19
合计	乡镇卫生院	1477	614	1	30.3	21
	社区卫生服务中心	1478	532	1	49.4	36
	小计	2955	614	1	39.8	28

2. 慢性病防控在岗人员年龄和工作经验

各级疾控中心慢性病防控在岗工作人员平均年龄为 38.4 岁，省、地市和县（区）三级差别不大，分别为 38.1 岁、40.0 岁和 38.1 岁。东、中、西部平均年龄差别也不大，分别为 37.0 岁、39.5 岁和 39.0 岁。从年龄段来看，全国范围内 35~44 岁组人员比例较高（35.1%），其次为 25~34 岁组（34.0%）。省级和地市级以 25~34 岁组构成比最高（分别为 45.0%和 32.6%），县（区）级以 35~44 岁组最高（36.8%）。

东部地区以 25~34 岁组构成比最高（41.8%），中、西部地区以 35~44 岁组构成比最高，分别为 35.9%和 37.3%。各级和不同地区疾控中心慢性病防控工作人员的年龄构成情况见图 2-3 和图 2-4。

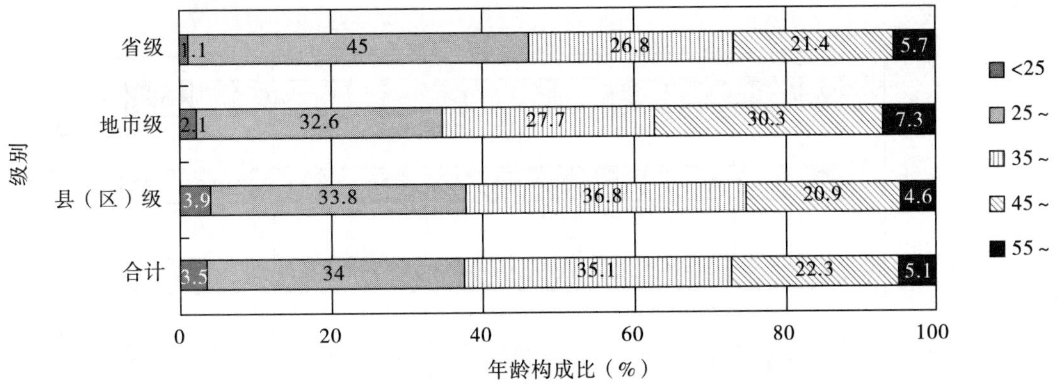

图 2-3 各级疾控中心慢性病防控人员的年龄构成比情况

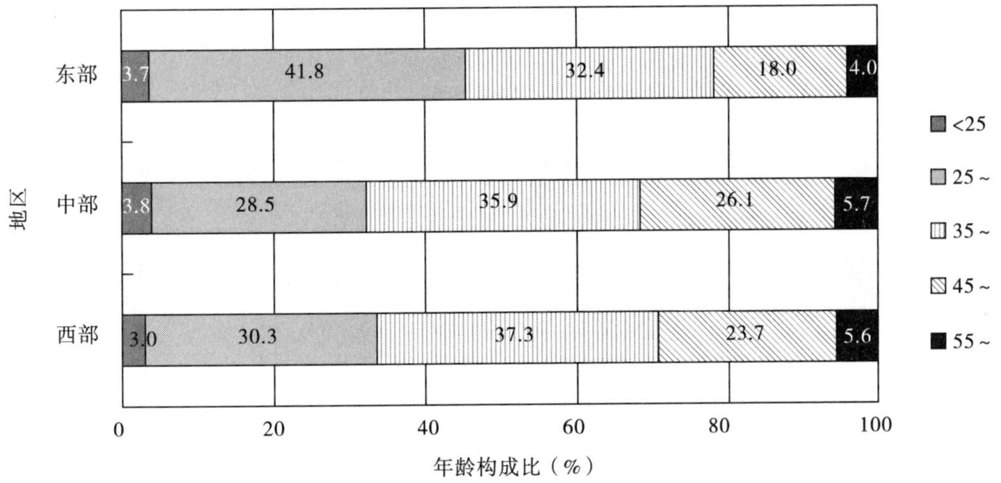

图 2-4 不同地区疾控中心慢性病防控工作人员的年龄构成情况

各级疾控中心慢性病防控在岗工作人员平均工作年限为 4.7 年，省、地市和县（区）三级依次下降，分别为 7.4 年、5.8 年和 4.4 年。东、中、西部地区工作年限依次下降，分别为 4.7 年、4.6 年和 4.1 年。全国范围内，66.6%的慢性病防控在岗人员工作年限不足 5 年。在省、地市、县（区）三级均以 5 年以下工作经验者为多，比例分别为 36.5%、52.3%和 70.6%。东、中、西部地区分布相似，均以 5 年以下工作经验者占绝大部分，比例分别为 59.8%、66.4%和 74.4%。各级和不同地区疾控中心慢性病防控工作人员的工作年限构成情况见图 2-5 和图 2-6。

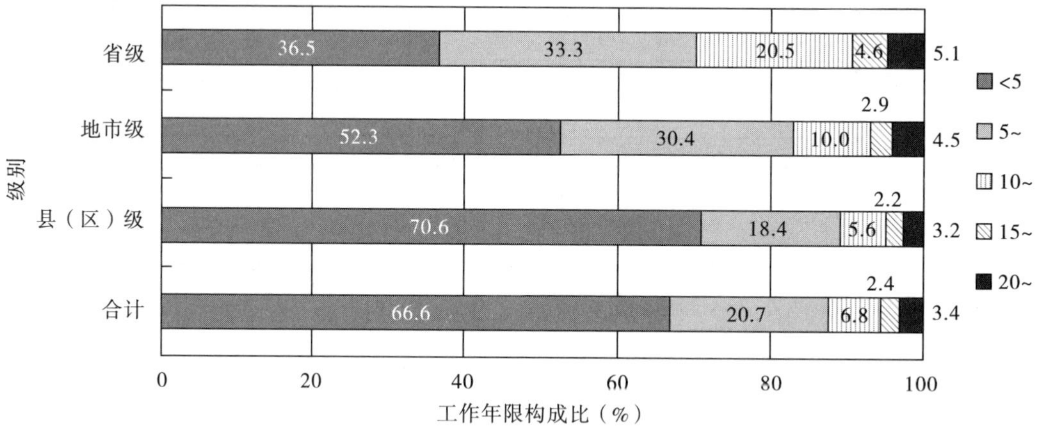

图 2-5 各级疾控中心慢性病防控工作人员的工作年限构成情况

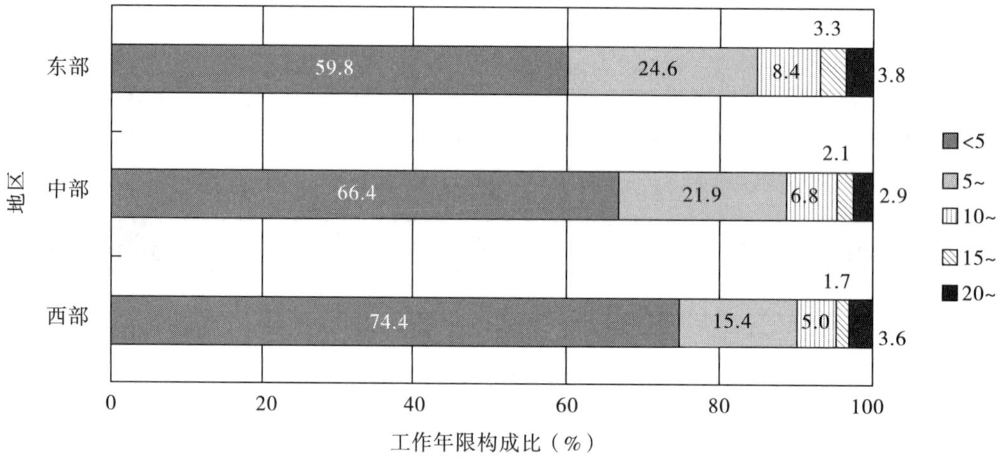

图 2-6 不同地区疾控中心慢性病防控工作人员的工作年限构成情况

3. 慢性病防控在岗人员学历

全国慢性病防控在岗人员中具有本科以上学历的比例为 43.7%，较 2009 年调查时（38.2%）有所增长，但仍有 18.7%的慢性病防控工作人员为中专及以下学历。各级疾控中心慢性病防控在岗人员中具有本科以上学历的比例按省、地市、县（区）三级呈现逐级下降，分别为 88.6%、64.1% 和 37.9%，均较 2009 年调查时（83.9%、59.2% 和

31.7%）有所增长。从地区分布来看，东部地区慢性病防控在岗人员中具有本科学历的比例最高，占45.8%，而中、西部地区则以具有大专学历的人员所占比重最大，分别为41.6%和44.7%。中、西部地区省和地市两级以本科学历比例为最高，县（区）级以大专比例最高；东部地区省级以硕士及以上比例最高，地市和县（区）两级以本科比例最高（图2-7和图2-8）。

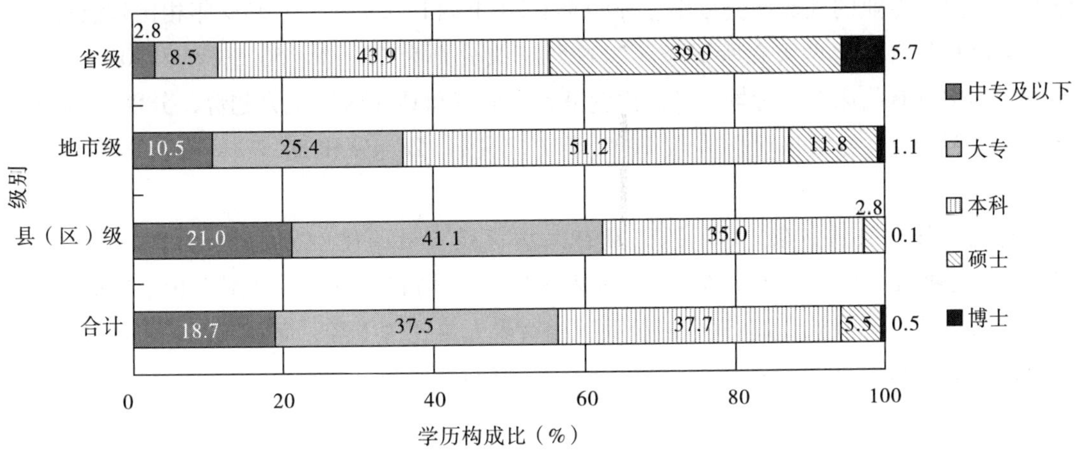

图2-7 各级疾控中心慢性病防控工作人员的学历构成情况

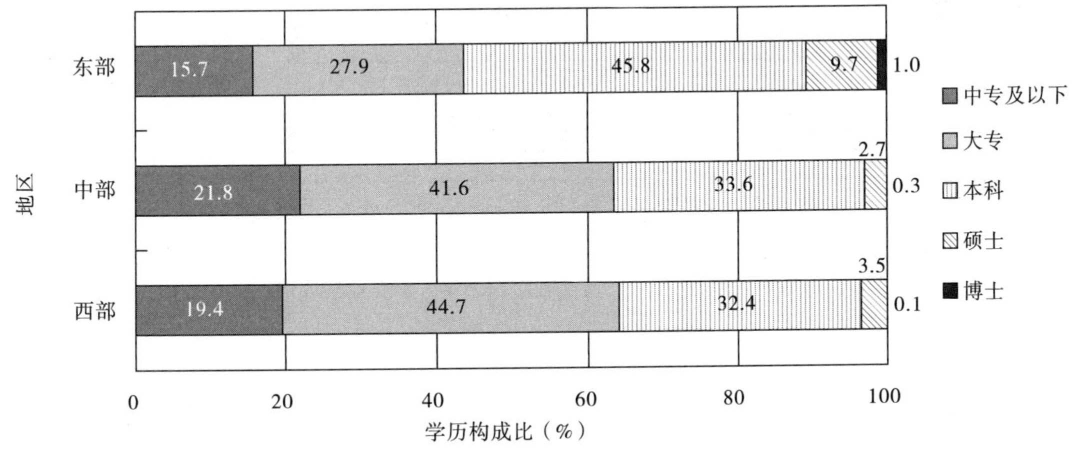

图2-8 不同地区疾控中心慢性病防控工作人员的学历构成情况

4. 慢性病防控在岗人员专业

本次调查中将慢性病防控在岗人员专业分为预防医学或公共卫生、临床医学、医学类其他专业、非医学类专业和无专业等 5 个类别。

全国疾控中心慢性病防控在岗人员中有医学专业背景的比例为 89.9%（2009 年为 91.4%），其中预防医学或公共卫生、临床医学为主要专业的比例分别为 40.1%和 30.1%，均较 2009 年（41.3%和 33%）有所下降。省、地市、县（区）三级疾控中心中具有预防医学或公共卫生专业的人员比例分别为 69.8%、50.4%和 36.9%，与 2009 年相比省级有所增加，地市和县（区）两级有所下降（2009 年三级分别为 67.4%、50.8%和 38.0%）；三级疾控中心中具有临床医学背景人员的比例呈省、地市和县（区）上升趋势，分别为 12.8%、26.4%和 31.6%，各级该比例均较 2009 年（17.4%、28.4%和 34.7%）有所下降（图 2-9）。

从地区分布来看，东、中、西部具有医学背景人员的比例分别为 90.5%、86.6%和 92.4%，各级较 2009 年（91.7%、89.3%和 93.8%）均有所下降，见图 2-10。各地区内也呈现出从省到县（区），预防医学或公共卫生背景人员比例下降，而临床医学背景人员比例上升的趋势，与 2009 年调查结果一致。

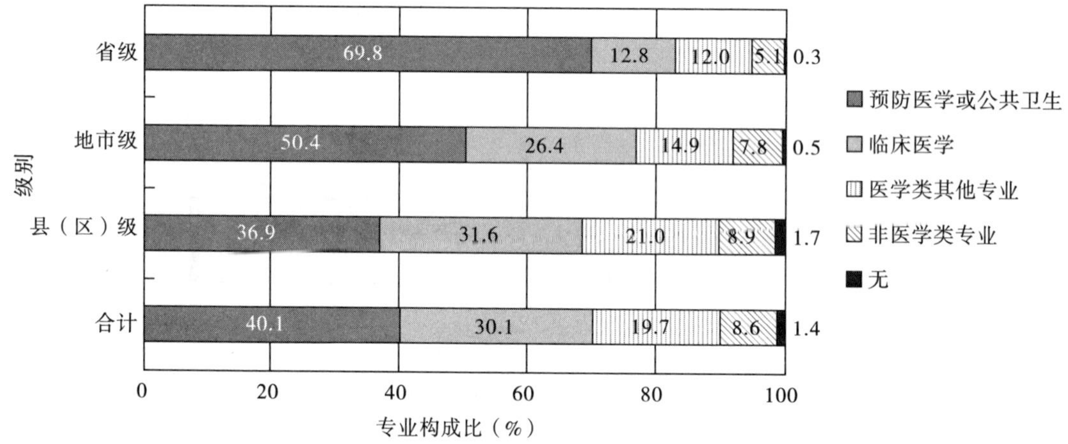

图 2-9 各级疾控中心慢性病防控工作人员专业构成情况

5. 慢性病防控在岗人员执业资格

对各地、各级疾控中心慢性病防控在岗工作人员取得执业资格（执业医师、助理医师、护士等）情况进行统计，应答的 9266 名慢性病防控在岗人员中 7150 名（77.2%）取得执业资格，省、地市和县（区）三级分别为 85.5%、85.6%和 75.2%。东、中、西部地区分别为 78.6%、73.1 和 79.2%（表 2-22）。

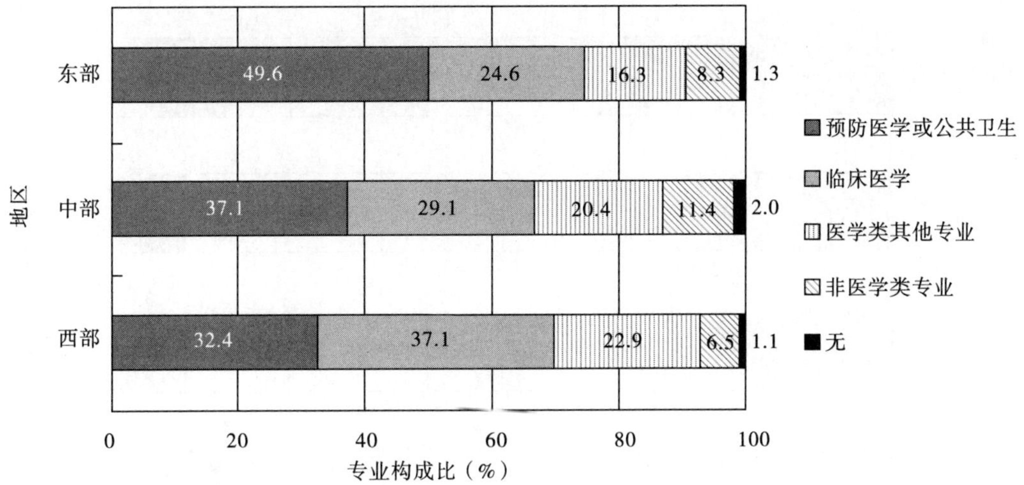

图 2-10　不同地区疾控中心慢性病防控工作人员专业构成情况

表 2-22　各地、各级疾控中心工作人员获得执业资格的情况［机构数（%）］

级别	东部	中部	西部	合计
省级	144（82.3）	62（83.8）	94（92.2）	300（85.5）
地市级	435（89.5）	360（84.3）	383（82.7）	1178（85.6）
县（区）级	2119（76.5）	1600（70.6）	1953（78.0）	5672（75.2）
合计	**2698（78.6）**	**2022（73.1）**	**2430（79.2）**	**7150（77.2）**

6. 慢性病防控在岗人员职称

全国慢性病防控工作人员中具有初级职称的比例最高为 38.9%，具有中级职称的占 36.6%，具有副高级职称的占 8.7%，具有正高级职称的占 2.3%。在省级和地市级疾控中心从事慢性病防控工作的人员中，具有中级职称的比例最高，分为占 37.9%和 38.1%，在县（区）级疾控中心从事慢性病防控工作的人员中，具有初级职称的比例最高，占 41.7%（图 2-11、图 2-12）。

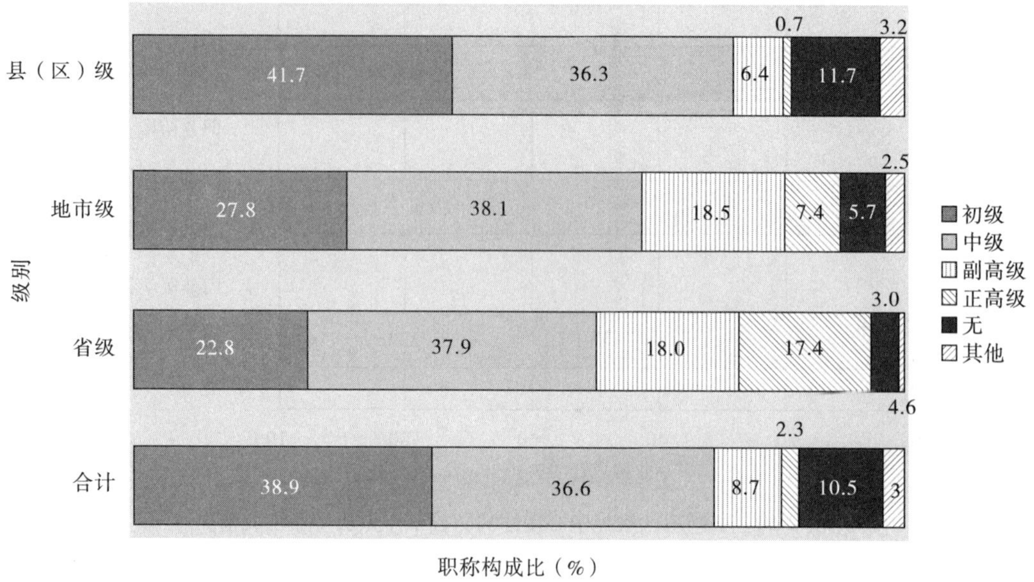

图 2-11　各级慢性病防控工作人员职称构成情况

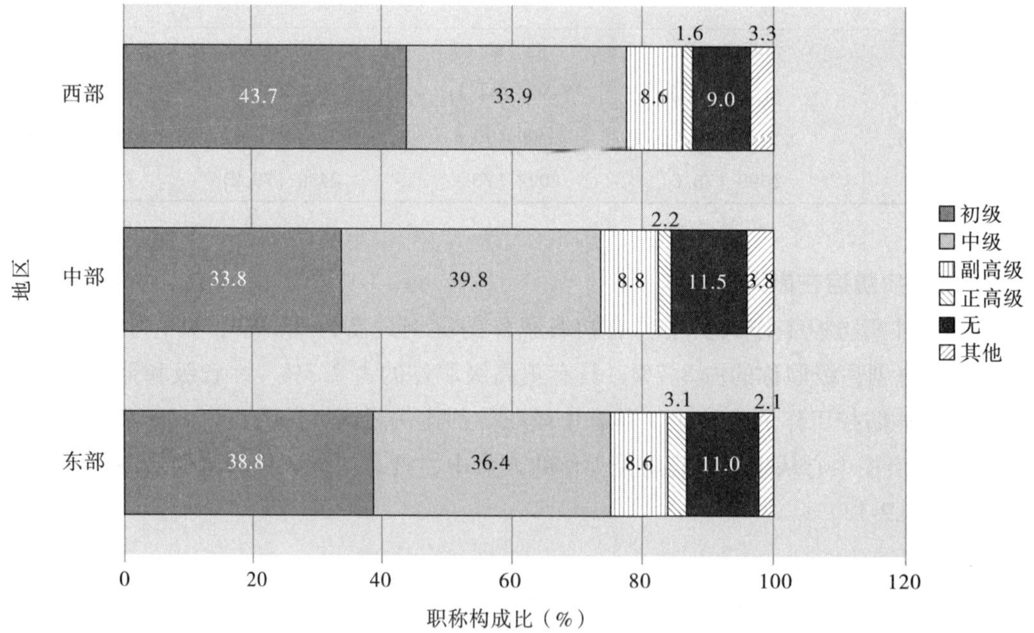

图 2-12　各地慢性病防控工作人员职称构成情况

（三）经费配置能力

经费配置能力主要指被调查疾控中心2011年到账的慢性病防控工作经费情况；被调查基层医疗卫生机构2011年到账的基本公共卫生服务经费情况。

（1）疾控中心

2011年，全国57.3%的疾控中心配置了慢性病防控工作经费，较2009年（40.2%）有较大增长，但低于2008年（71.5%）；其中省、地市、县（区）三级该比例分别为96.9%、76.0%和54.6%，与2009年（100%、55.7%和37.4%）相比，除省级有所降低外，地市、县（区）两级均有增加。东、中、西部地区疾控中心配置慢性病防控工作经费的比例依次为66.0%、56.3%和51.5%，各地区内也呈现省、地市、县（区）逐级下降的趋势。东部地区各级疾控中心经费配置情况均好于中部和西部地区，西部县（区）级配置经费的机构比例最低（48.5%），但较2009年（仅26.2%）有所增长（表2-23和图2-13）。

表2-23　各地、各级疾控中心配置慢性病防控工作经费情况［机构数（%）］

级别	东部	中部	西部	合计
省级	11（100.0）	8（100.0）	12（92.3）	31（96.9）
地市级	86（87.8）	73（70.2）	104（72.2）	263（76.0）
县（区）级	558（63.1）	479（54.2）	568（48.5）	1605（54.6）
合计	**655（66.0）**	**560（56.3）**	**684（51.5）**	**1899（57.3）**

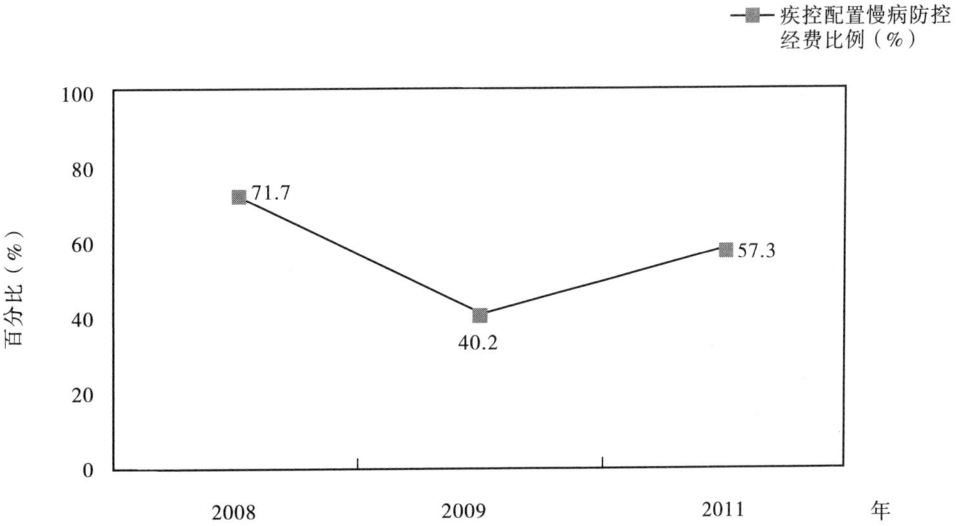

图2-13　全国疾控中心配置慢性病防控经费比例变化图

省、地市、县（区）三级疾控中心慢性病防控工作经费依次平均为 181.6 万元、17.0 万元和 13.7 万元，均较 2009 年（分别为 147.7 万元、14.2 万元和 9.1 万元）和 2008 年（分别为 86.3 万元、8.9 万元和 4.5 万元）明显增加，但地市和县（区）两级经费虽呈增长趋势，但与省级相比经费差距仍较大（表 2-24 和图 2-14）。

表 2-24　各级疾控中心配置慢性病防控工作经费情况（万元，人民币）

级别	最大值	最小值	平均数	中位数
省级	1329.8	30.5	181.6	80.0
地市级	641.5	0.2	17.0	5.0
县（区）级	655.0	0.1	13.7	4.7
合计	1329.9	0.1	16.9	5.0

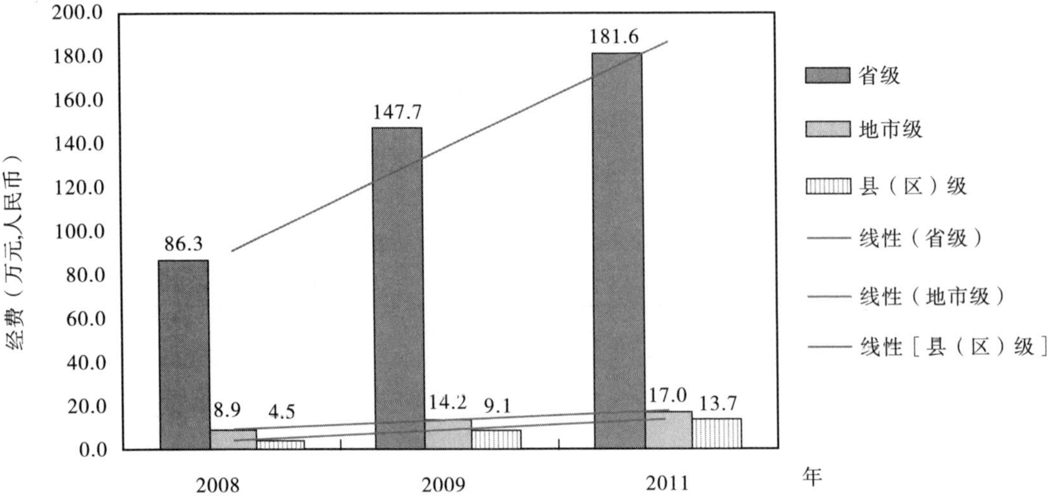

图 2-14　各级疾控中心配置慢性病防控工作经费变化图

全国省级疾控中心慢性病防控工作经费以东部地区某省最高，达 1329.9 万元，中部地区某省经费最低（仅 30.5 万元），但相比 2009 年调查时西部某省 1.7 万元的最低值有较大提高。从地区分布来看，东部地区各级疾控中心慢性病防控工作经费的平均数和中位数均高于中、西部地区（表 2-25）。

表 2-25 不同地区疾控中心配置慢性病防控工作经费情况（万元，人民币）

地区	最大值	最小值	平均数	中位数
东部	1329.9	0.1	26.3	7.0
中部	297	0.1	10.8	3.0
西部	208.4	0.1	12.75	4.0
合计	1329.9	0.1	16.9	5.0

全国各地各级疾控中心的慢性病防控工作经费占疾控中心业务经费比例为4.4%，较2009年（2.7%）有所增长。省、地市和县（区）三级分别为2.0%、3.1%和7.4%，地市、县（区）两级较2009年（2.2%和2.9%）和2008年（1.7%和2.7%）有所增加，其中县（区）级增长幅度最大（图2-15）。

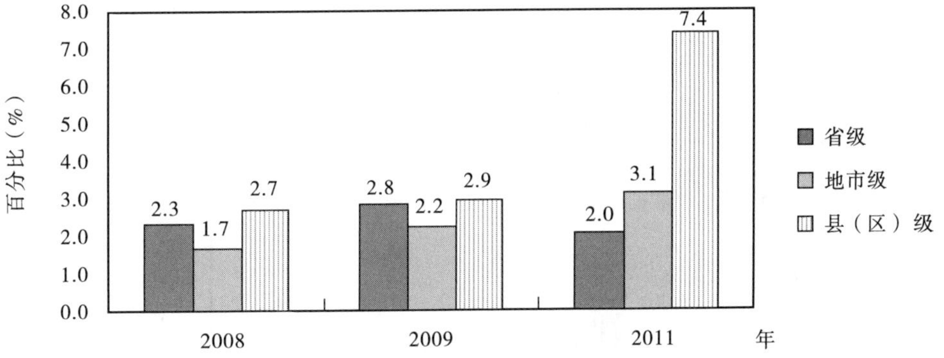

图2-15 各级疾控中心配置慢性病防控工作经费占疾控中心业务经费变化图

东、中、西部地区疾控中心慢性病防控经费占疾控中心业务经费的比例分别依次为5.0%、4.3%和3.6%，均较2009年（2.6%、3.7%和2.0%）有所增长；东部地区的省级和地市级疾控中心慢性病防控工作经费占疾控中心业务经费的比例均高于中、西部地区，而县（区）级这一比例则以西部地区最高（7.9%）（表2-26）。

表 2-26 不同地区疾控中心配置慢性病防控工作经费占疾控业务经费比例（%）

级别	东部	中部	西部	合计
省级	2.8	1.9	1.0	2.0
地市级	4.6	1.6	2.4	3.1

续 表

级别	东部	中部	西部	合计
县（区）级	7.2	7.3	7.9	7.4
合计	5.0	4.3	3.6	4.4

（2）基层医疗卫生机构

在应答的 2955 家基层医疗卫生机构中，有 2822 家在 2011 年获得了基本公共卫生服务经费，占 95.5%；获得基本公共卫生服务经费的平均数额为 85.4 万元，其中乡镇卫生院平均数额为 52.4 万元，社区卫生服务中心平均数额为 117.9 万元。东、中、西部地区基本公共卫生服务经费的平均数额分别为 128.3 万元、63.6 万元和 53.9 万元，中、西部较东部有较大差距。被调查基层医疗卫生服务机构获得基本公共卫生服务经费的最高额达 1448.9 万元，最低仅为 1000 元（图 2-16）。

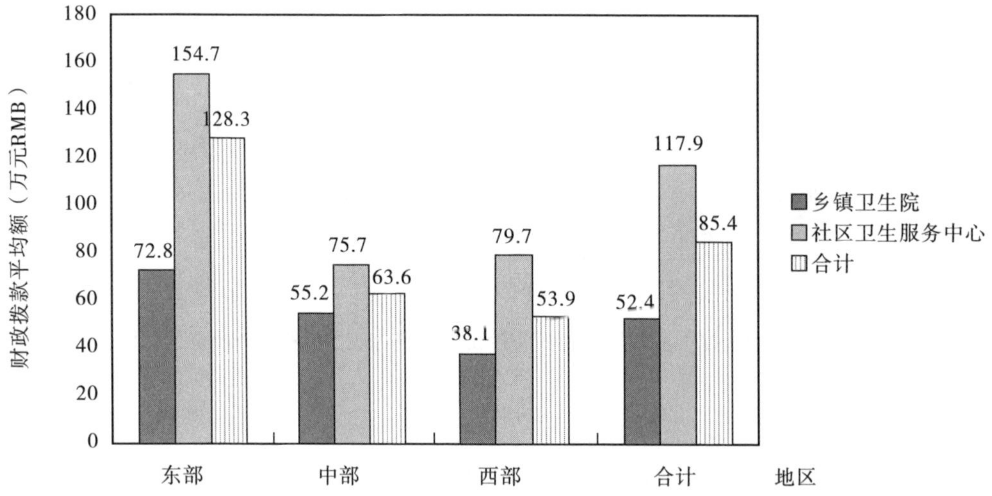

图 2-16 各地基层医疗卫生机构基本公共卫生服务经费平均数额情况

2011 年，在应答的 2955 家基层医疗卫生机构中，共有 2881 家有到账的财政拨款，占 97.5%。财政拨款平均 245.3 万元，其中乡镇卫生院平均 142.5 万元，社区卫生服务中心平均 347.4 万元。东、中、西部基层医疗卫生机构获得财政拨款的平均数额依次为 405.3 万元、149.4 万元和 138.9 万元，中、西部地区较东部地区有较大差距。被调查的基层医疗卫生机构获得财政拨款最多 9308 万元，最低仅为 2000 元（图 2-17）。

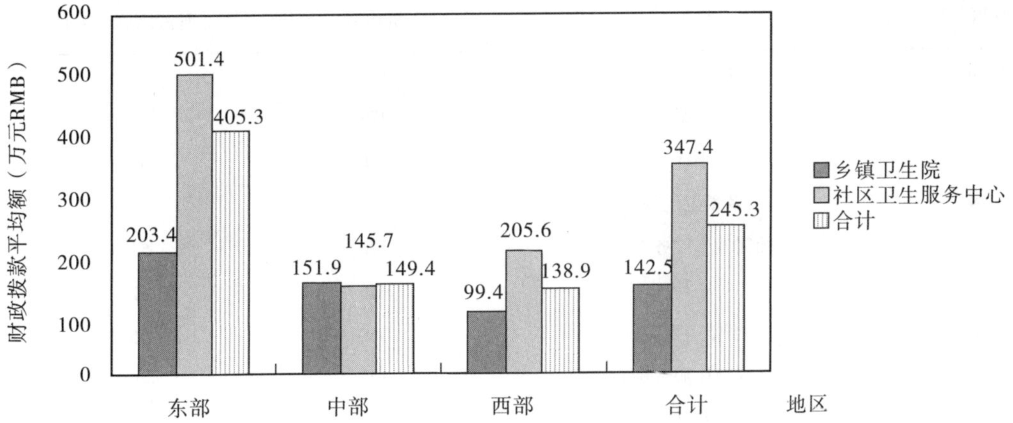

图 2-17　各地基层医疗卫生机构平均财政拨款平均数额情况

在获得基本公共卫生服务经费的 2822 家基层医疗卫生机构中，34. 8%的财政拨款来源于基本公共卫生服务经费，较 2009 年有所下降（37. 6%）；其中乡镇卫生院为 36. 3%，社区卫生服务中心为 34. 1%。这一比例在中部地区最高，为 42. 4%，其中又以中部地区社区卫生服务中心的比例最高，达 51. 8%，东部和西部地区分别为 31. 8%和 37. 9%（图 2-18）。

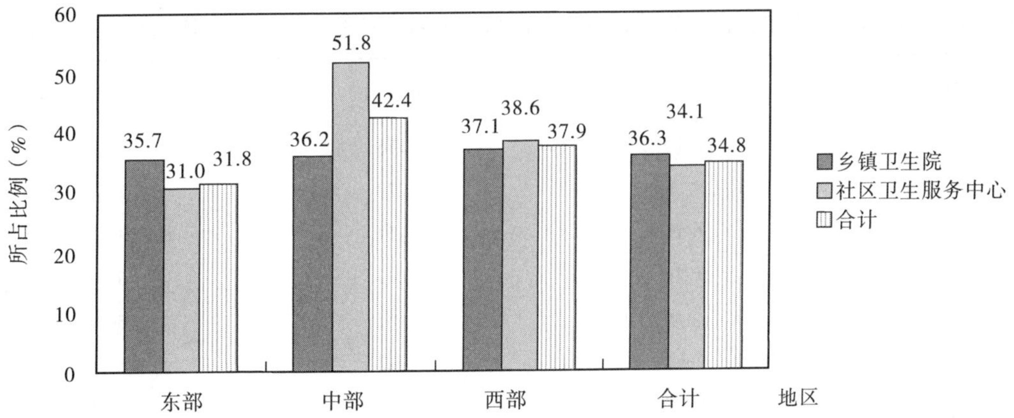

图 2-18　各地基层医疗卫生机构基本公共卫生服务经费占 2011 年到账财政拨款的比例

本次调查中有 1405（47. 5%）家基层医疗卫生机构回答有针对高血压患者管理工作进行费用核算，乡镇卫生院和社区卫生服务中心该比例分别为 53. 0%和 42. 1%，东、中、西部地区该比例依次为 39. 9%、52. 1%和 52. 6%，中、西部高于东部（表 2-27）。

表 2-27　各地基层医疗卫生机构所在县（区）针对高血压病例管理设置单项财政经费补助情况

地区	机构	机构数	所占比例（%）
东部	乡镇卫生院	177	47.6
	社区卫生服务中心	279	36.2
	小计	456	39.9
中部	乡镇卫生院	246	52.7
	社区卫生服务中心	170	51.4
	小计	416	52.1
西部	乡镇卫生院	360	56.4
	社区卫生服务中心	173	46.0
	小计	533	52.6
合计	乡镇卫生院	783	53.0
	社区卫生服务中心	622	42.1
	小计	1405	47.5

本次调查中有 1397（47.3%）家基层医疗卫生机构回答有针对糖尿病患者管理工作进行费用核算，乡镇卫生院和社区卫生服务中心该比例分别为 52.7%和 41.9%，东、中、西部地区该比例依次为 39.7%、51.6%和 52.4%，中、西部明显高于东部（表 2-28）。

表 2-28　各地基层医疗卫生机构所在县（区）针对糖尿病病例管理项目设置单项财政经费补助情况

地区	机构类型	机构数	所占比例（%）
东部	乡镇卫生院	176	47.3
	社区卫生服务中心	278	36.1
	小计	454	39.7
中部	乡镇卫生院	245	52.5
	社区卫生服务中心	167	50.5
	小计	412	51.6
西部	乡镇卫生院	357	56.0
	社区卫生服务中心	174	46.3
	小计	531	52.4
合计	乡镇卫生院	778	52.7
	社区卫生服务中心	619	41.9
	小计	1397	47.3

（四）设备配置能力

设备配置能力主要指基层医疗卫生机构配置慢性病防控相关设备的情况。

调查发现，基层医疗卫生机构配备体重秤、身高计、腰围尺、血压计、血糖仪的比例均在90%以上，其次为心电图机（82.8%）、B超（79.5%）、生化仪（72.1%）、健教设备（71.9%）和X线机（66.8%），配备肺功能仪的比例最低仅为16.3%（图2-19）。社区卫生服务中心配置各类设备的比例较2009年变化不大，乡镇卫生院配置各类设备的比例较2009年有大幅度增加。2011年乡镇卫生院配备体重秤、身高计、腰围尺、血压计的比例均达到90%以上，而2009年的配置比例仅为70%～80%，健教设备的配置比例更是从2009年的29%增加到60.9%（图2-20、图2-21）。

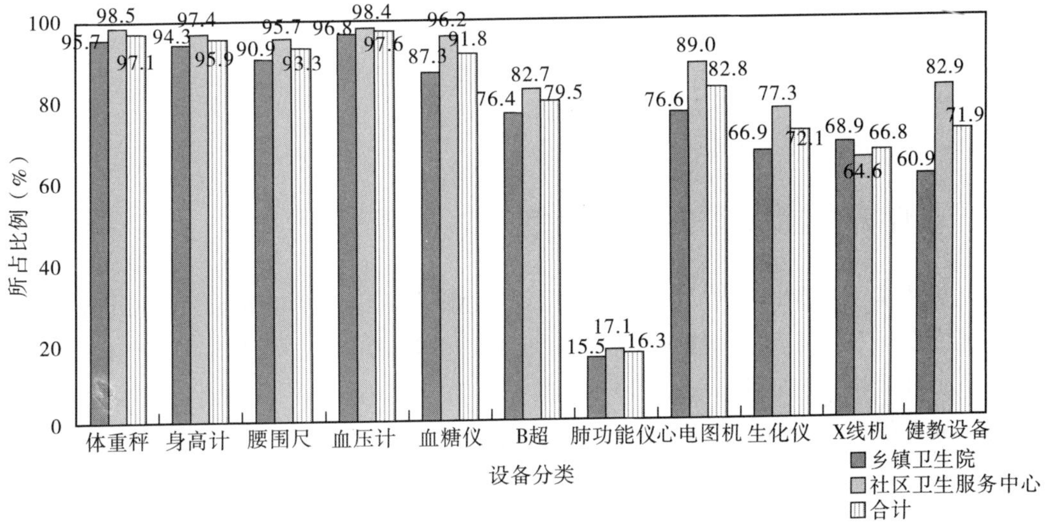

图2-19 全国基层医疗卫生机构配置各类慢性病防控相关设备的情况

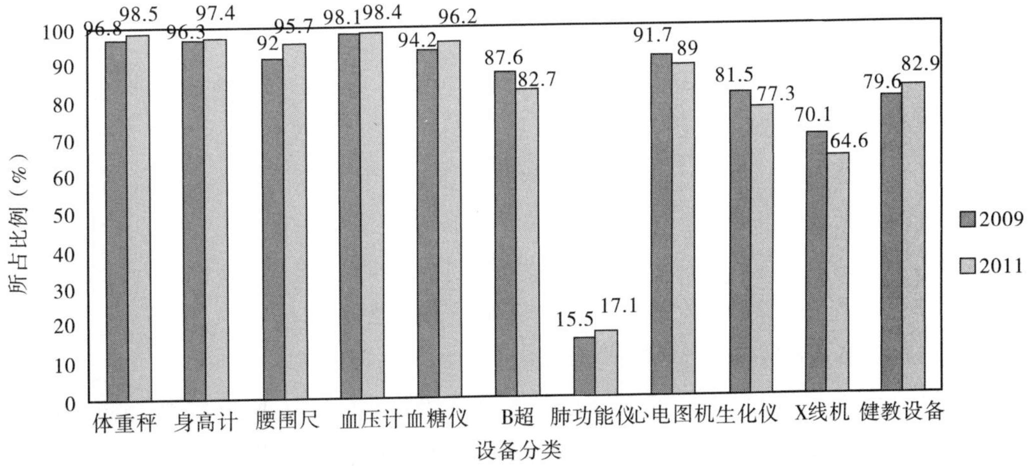

图2-20 2009和2011年社区卫生服务中心配置各类慢性病防控相关设备变化图

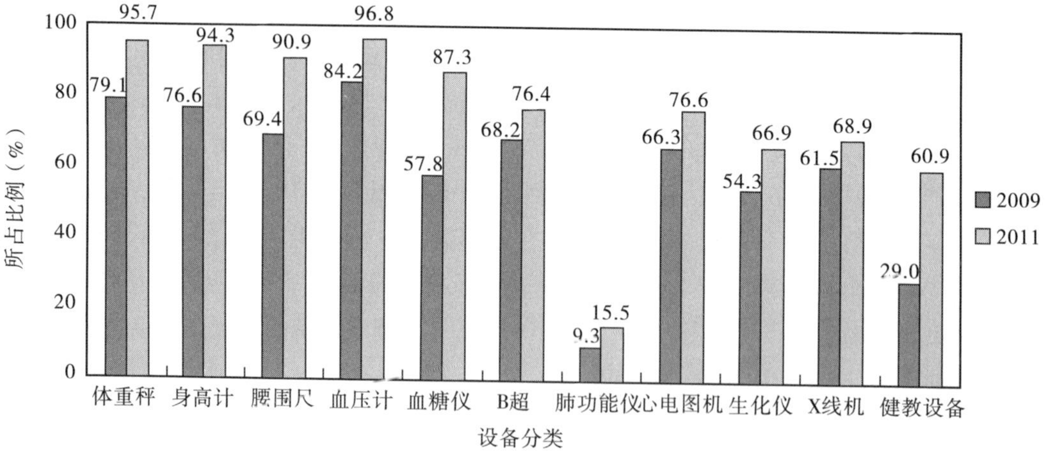

图 2-21　2009 和 2011 年乡镇卫生院配置各类慢性病防控相关设备变化图

四、慢性病防控教育培训与指导能力

慢性病防控教育培训与指导能力是一个广义的概念，它包括培训能力、指导能力和知识普及能力等三个方面。培训能力：包括开展培训和参与培训。开展培训，即对慢性病防控工作人员开展相关培训的情况；参与培训，即组织本单位人员参与慢性病防控相关培训的情况。指导能力：即对下级机构开展慢性病防控工作现场指导的情况。知识普及能力：主要指基层医疗卫生机构将慢性病防控相关知识传播给大众的情况。

（一）培训能力

1. 组织开展培训情况

2011 年全国各级疾控中心有 2227 家机构举办过各类慢性病防控相关培训班，比例为 67. 2%，(2009 年为 43. 5%)，其中东部、中部、西部地区各级疾控中心举办各类相关培训的比例分别为 79. 8%、63. 5%、60. 5%，省级、地市级、县（区）级疾控中心举办各类相关培训的比例分别为 100. 0%、70. 5%、66. 4% [2009 年省、地市、县（区）比例分别为 96. 9%、50. 3%、42. 1%]，同一地区不同级别的疾控中心举办各类培训班的比例从省级到县（区）级总体呈递降趋势，趋势与 2009 年一致（图 2-22）。

（1）各地、各级疾控中心举办各类慢性病防控相关培训班情况

2011 年，全国有 30 个省级疾控中心举办了省级培训班，占所有省级机构的比例为 93. 8%（比例与 2009 年一致）；221 个地市级疾控中心举办了地市级培训班，占地市级机构的比例为 63. 9%（2009 年为 44. 8%）；县（区）级疾控中心举办县（区）级培训班的机构

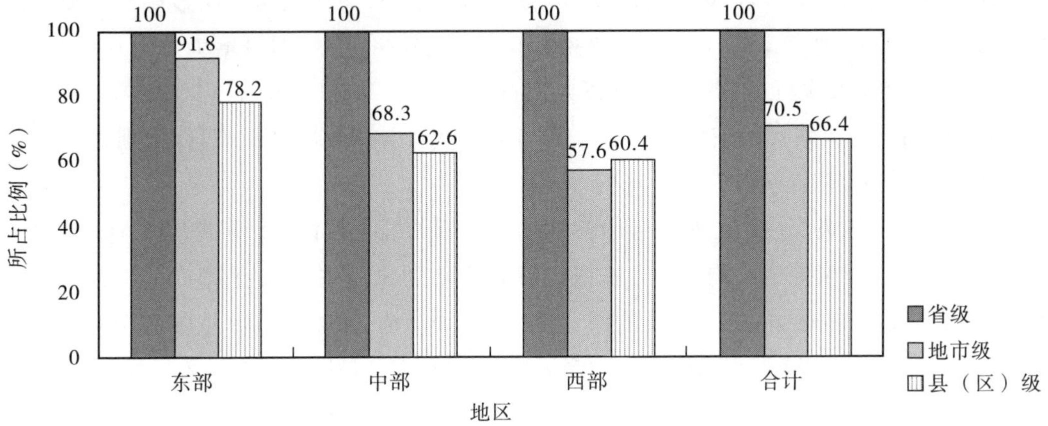

图 2-22 各地、各级疾控中心举办慢性病防控相关培训班的情况

数最多，为 1928 个，所占比例为 65.6%（2009 年为 40.0%）。全国仅西部 2 个县（区）级（0.07%）疾控中心举办过国际级培训班，省、地市、县（区）分别有 5 个（15.6%）、14 个（4.0%）和 27 个（0.9%）机构举办过国家级培训班。从地区分布来看，各疾控中心举办省级培训班的比例西部略高于东、中部地区，而举办国家级、地市级和县（区）级培训班的机构比例东部均高于中、西部地区（表 2-29、表 2-30）。

表 2-29 全国各级疾控中心举办慢性病防控相关培训班的情况［机构数（%）］

级别	培训班类别				
	国际级	国家级	省级	地市级	县（区）级
省级	0（0.0）	5（15.6）	30（93.8）	1（3.1）	4（12.5）
地市级	0（0.0）	14（4.0）	18（5.2）	221（63.9）	46（13.3）
县（区）级	2（0.07）	27（0.9）	40（1.4）	64（2.2）	1928（65.6）
合计	**2（0.06）**	**46（1.4）**	**88（2.7）**	**286（8.6）**	**1978（59.7）**

表 2-30 全国各地疾控中心举办慢性病防控相关培训班的情况［机构数（%）］

地区	培训班类别				
	国际级	国家级	省级	地市级	县（区）级
东部	0（0.0）	18（1.8）	26（2.6）	104（10.5）	700（70.5）
中部	0（0.0）	15（1.5）	25（2.5）	82（8.2）	562（56.5）
西部	2（0.15）	13（1.0）	37（2.8）	100（7.5）	716（54.0）
合计	**2（0.06）**	**46（1.4）**	**88（2.7）**	**286（8.6）**	**1978（59.7）**

2011 年，全国各级慢性病防控相关培训班共培训 298 273 人次，明显高于 2009 年的 163 972人次。省、地市、县（区）三级疾控中心开展的各级培训班培训总人次数逐级增多，分别为 2554 人次（0.9%）、11 328人次（3.8%）、284 391人次（95.3%）。东、中、西部地区培训总人次数，以东部最多，为114 165人次（38.3%），中、西部分别为86 329人次（28.9%）、97 779人次（32.8%）。

（2）各地、各级疾控中心举办各级慢性病防控相关继续教育培训班情况

2011 年，各级疾控中心均以举办本级继续教育培训班为主，其中 22 个省级疾控中心、91 个地市级疾控中心举办了本级的继续教育培训。省、地市、县（区）分别有 5 个（15.6%）、10 个（2.9%）和24 个（0.8%）疾控中心举办过国家级继续教育培训。从地区分布来看，除举办国家级继续教育培训班的机构比例呈东、中、西递减的趋势外，举办省级和地市级的机构比例均是东、西、中部递减（表 2-31 和表 2-32）。

表 2-31　各级疾控中心举办慢性病防控相关继续教育培训班的情况［机构数（%）］

级别	继续教育分类		
	国家级	省级	地市级
省级	5（15.6）	22（68.8）	0（0.0）
地市级	10（2.9）	15（4.3）	91（26.3）
县（区）级	24（0.8）	22（0.7）	27（0.9）
合计	**39（1.2）**	**59（1.8）**	**118（3.6）**

表 2-32　各地疾控中心举办慢性病防控相关继续教育培训班的情况［机构数（%）］

地区	继续教育分类		
	国家级	省级	地市级
东部	17（1.7）	22（2.2）	59（5.9）
中部	13（1.3）	15（1.5）	23（2.3）
西部	9（0.7）	22（1.7）	36（2.7）
合计	**39（1.2）**	**59（1.8）**	**118（3.6）**

（3）基层医疗卫生机构举办培训情况

2011 年，有 2437 个基层医疗卫生机构举办了慢性病防控相关培训班，占被调查基层医疗卫生机构的 82.5%（2009 年为 58.8%），其中社区卫生服务中心 1200 家，占被调查同类机构的 81.2%（2009 年为 72.5%），乡镇卫生院 1237 个，占被调查同类机构的 83.8%（2009 年为 44.6%）。从地区分布来看，举办慢性病相关培训班的基层医疗卫生机构比例以中部最高（85.1%），其次分别为东部（85.0%）和西部（77.5%）。所有地区乡镇卫生院

举办培训的机构比例均高于社区卫生服务中心（图 2-23）。

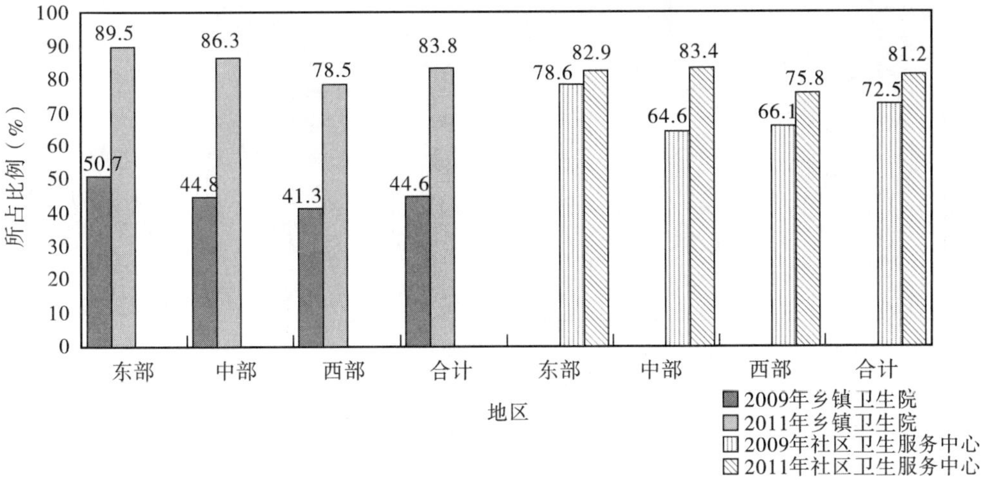

图 2-23　2009、2011 年举办慢性病防控相关培训班的各地基层医疗卫生机构的情况

2011 年各地基层医疗卫生机构举办培训班的平均次数为 4. 5 次，平均人次数为 242. 7 人次，最多举办培训班 48 次，培训 8856 人次。从地区分布来看，东部基层医疗卫生机构平均举办培训班 4. 7 次，平均培训 268. 4 人次，中部平均举办培训班 4. 5 次，平均培训 232. 1 人次，西部平均举办培训班 4. 2 次，平均培训 220. 1 人次（图 2-24、图 2-25）。

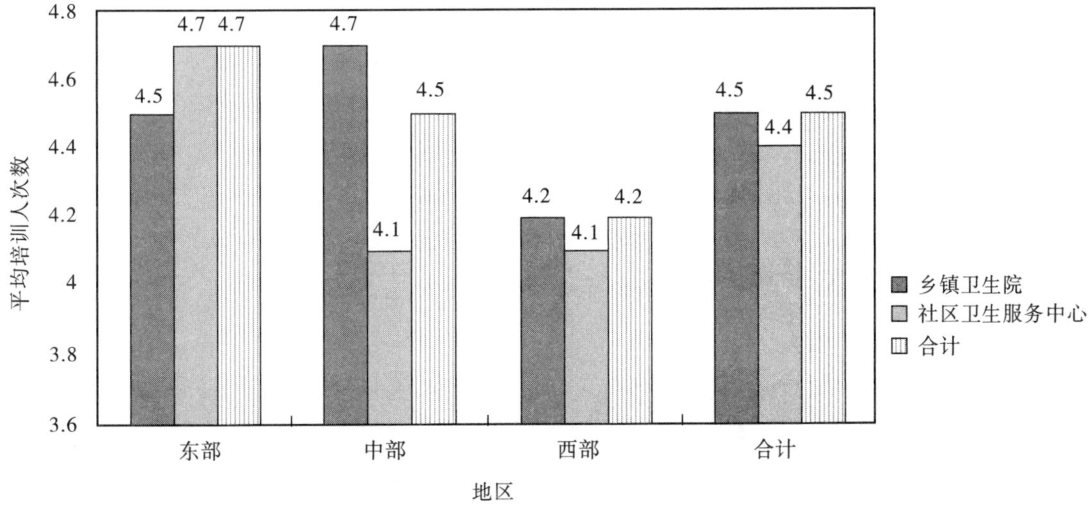

图 2-24　各地基层医疗卫生机构平均举办慢性病防控相关培训班的次数情况

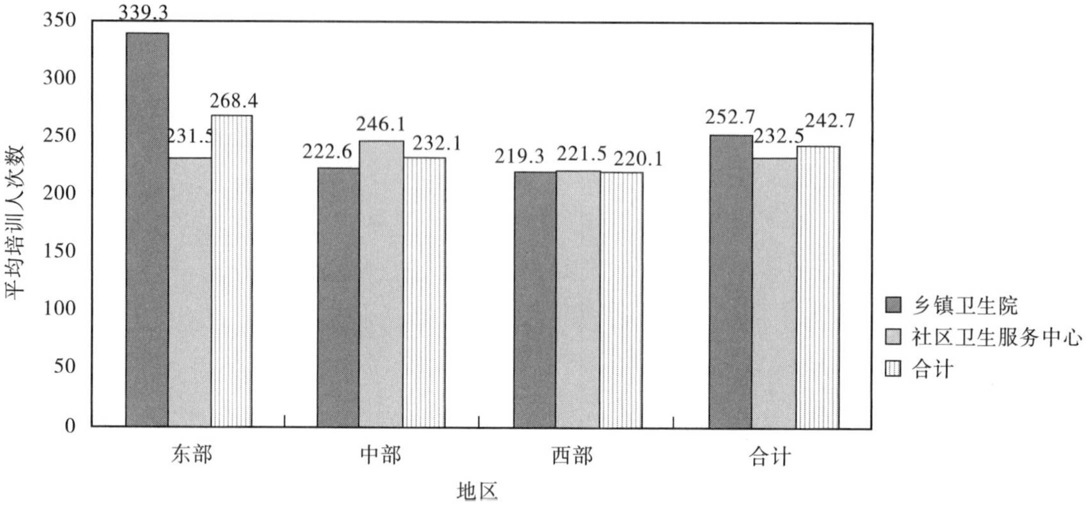

图 2-25 各地基层医疗卫生机构平均举办慢性病防控相关培训班的人次数情况

2. 各类培训参加情况

2011 年，全国共有 2603 个疾控中心派人员参加了各类慢性病防控相关培训班，占被调查疾控中心的 78.5%，(2009 年为 53.8%)。省、地市、县（区）级疾控中心派人员参加培训班的机构比例逐级降低，分别为 93.8%、89.0%、77.1% （2009 年分别为 96.9%、72.5%和 51.1%)。从地区分布看，东、中、西部疾控中心派人员参加培训班的机构比例依次降低，分别为 90.6%、83.7%和 65.6%（2009 年分别为 69.6%、61.2%和 36%)。各地区省、地市、县（区）级疾控中心派人员参加培训班的机构比例逐级下降（图 2-26)。

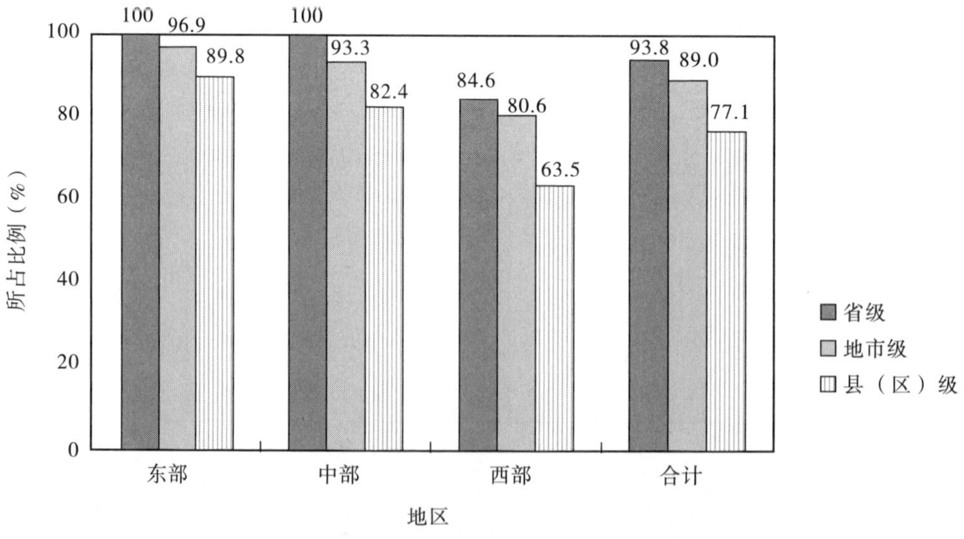

图 2-26 各地、各级疾控中心派人员参加慢性病防控相关培训班的情况

(1) 各地、各级疾控中心派人员参加各级慢性病防控相关培训班的情况

2011 年，全国有 30 个省级疾控中心派人员参加过国家级培训班，比例为 93.8%；地市级疾控中心以派人员参加省级培训班的机构数量最多，为 299 个，所占比例为 86.4%；县（区）级疾控中心以派人员参加地市级培训班的机构数量最多，为 1593 个，所占比例为 54.2%。各级疾控中心派人员参加慢性病防控培训班的比例以参加省级培训班的比例最高，占 54.6%，各级参加国际级、国家级、地市级和县（区）级的比例分别为 0.7%、9.9%、50.9%和 25.8%。从地区分布来看，除省级培训班外，参加国际级、国家级、地市级和县（区）级慢性病防控相关培训班的机构比例均呈东、中、西部递减的趋势（表 2-33、表 2-34）。

表 2-33 各级疾控中心派人员参加慢性病防控相关培训班的情况 [机构数（%）]

级别	培训班类别				
	国际级	国家级	省级	地市级	县（区）级
省级	9（28.1）	30（93.8）	16（50.0）	1（3.1）	2（6.3）
地市级	10（2.9）	81（23.4）	299（86.4）	93（26.9）	14（4.0）
县（区）级	5（0.2）	216（7.4）	1496（50.9）	1593（54.2）	839（28.6）
合计	**24（0.7）**	**327（9.9）**	**1811（54.6）**	**1687（50.9）**	**855（25.8）**

表 2-34 各地区疾控中心派人员参加慢性病防控相关培训班的情况 [机构数（%）]

地区	培训班类别				
	国际级	国家级	省级	地市级	县（区）级
东部	13（1.3）	147（14.8）	545（54.9）	675（68.0）	298（30.0）
中部	6（0.6）	90（9.0）	689（69.2）	487（48.9）	257（25.8）
西部	5（0.4）	90（6.8）	577（43.5）	525（39.6）	300（22.6）
合计	**24（0.7）**	**327（9.9）**	**1811（54.6）**	**1687（50.9）**	**855（25.8）**

(2) 各地、各级疾控中心派人参加各级慢性病防控相关继续教育培训班的情况

2011 年，有 18 个省级疾控中心派人员参加国家级继续教育培训班，占机构比例的 56.3%；地市级疾控中心以派人员参加省级继续教育培训班的机构数量最多，为 183 个，所占比例为 52.9%；县（区）级疾控中心以派人员参加省级继续教育培训班的机构数量最多，为 827 个，所占比例为 28.2%。从地区分布来看，除国际级继续教育培训外，派人员参加国家级、省级和地市级慢性病防控相关继续培训班的机构比例均呈东、中、西部递减的趋势（表 2-35、表 2-36）。

表 2-35 各级疾控中心派人员参加慢性病防控继续教育培训班的情况 [机构数 (%)]

级别	继续教育分类			
	国际级	国家级	省级	地市级
省级	1 (3.1)	18 (56.3)	13 (40.6)	1 (3.1)
地市级	3 (0.9)	38 (11.0)	183 (52.9)	44 (12.7)
县（区）级	1 (0.03)	129 (4.4)	827 (28.2)	556 (18.9)
合计	5 (0.2)	185 (5.6)	1023 (30.9)	601 (18.1)

表 2-36 各地疾控中心派人员参加慢性病防控继续教育培训班的情况 [机构数 (%)]

地区	继续教育分类			
	国际级	国家级	省级	地市级
东部	4 (0.4)	95 (9.6)	386 (38.9)	270 (27.2)
中部	0 (0.0)	44 (4.4)	350 (35.2)	166 (16.7)
西部	1 (0.1)	46 (3.5)	287 (21.6)	165 (12.4)
合计	5 (0.2)	185 (5.6)	1023 (30.9)	601 (18.1)

（3）基层医疗卫生机构参加慢性病防控相关培训的情况

2011 年，被调查基层医疗卫生机构中，共有 2651 个基层医疗卫生机构派人员参加了慢性病防控相关培训班，所占比例为 89.7%，（2009 年为 68.3%），其中社区卫生服务中心 1382 个，乡镇卫生院 1269 个，所占比例分别为 93.5%和 85.9%，与 2009 年时所占比例 84.7%和 51.3%相比均有明显增加。各地区被调查社区卫生服务中心参加慢性病防控相关培训班的比例均高于乡镇卫生院（图 2-27）。

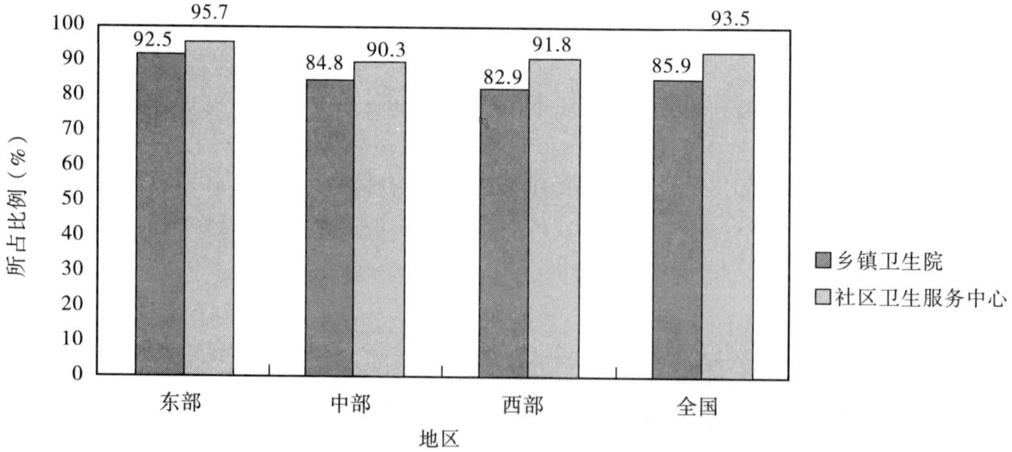

图 2-27 各地基层医疗卫生机构组织人员参加慢性病防控相关培训班的情况

2011年，在派人员参加慢性病防控相关培训班的基层医疗卫生服务机构中，以参加疾控中心举办培训班的比例最高，占79.5%，其中社区卫生服务中心为86.7%、乡镇卫生院为72.2%；其次是卫生行政部门，比例为65.0%，其中社区卫生服务中心为66.6%、乡镇卫生院为63.3%；再次是医院，比例为37.1%，其中社区卫生服务中心为45.0%、乡镇卫生院为29.2%；参加其他机构或部门举办的培训班比例为14.9%，其中社区卫生服务中心为19.9%，乡镇卫生院为9.8%。

社区卫生服务中心派人员参加各类部门举办的培训班的平均人数和平均人次数均高于乡镇卫生院，乡镇卫生院和社区卫生服务中心参加医院举办的培训班的平均次数和平均人次数均高于参加其他机构举办的培训班（图2-28、图2-29和图2-30）。

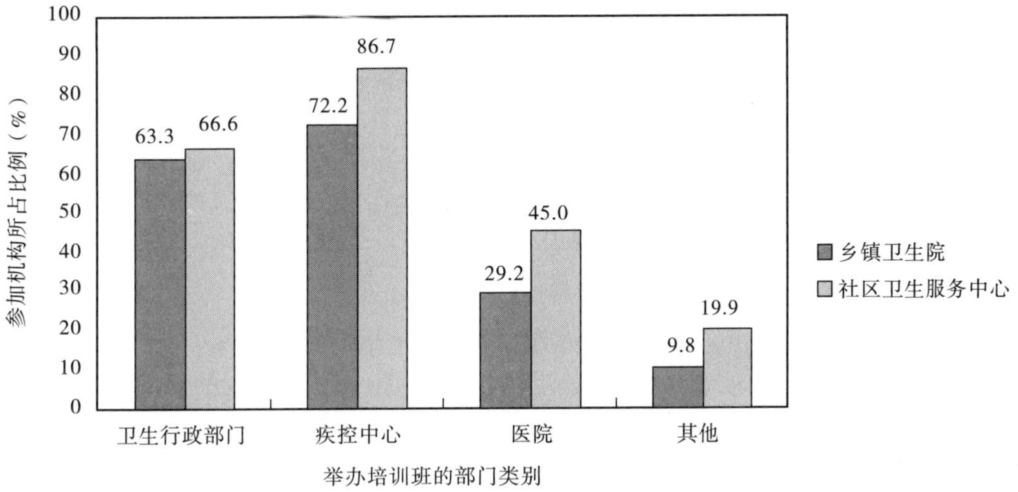

图2-28　基层医疗卫生机构组织人员参加各类机构举办的慢性病防控相关培训班的比例

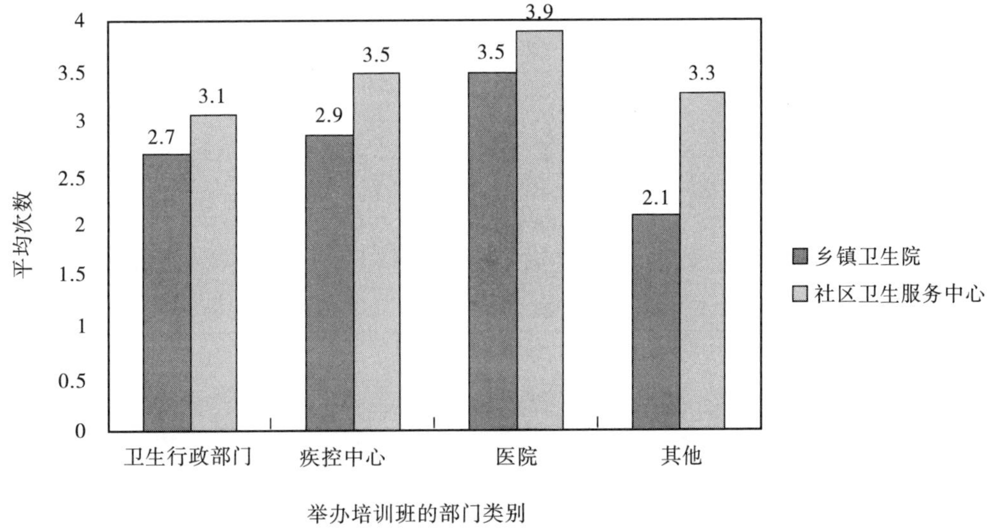

图2-29　基层医疗卫生机构组织人员参加各类机构举办的慢性病防控相关培训班的平均次数

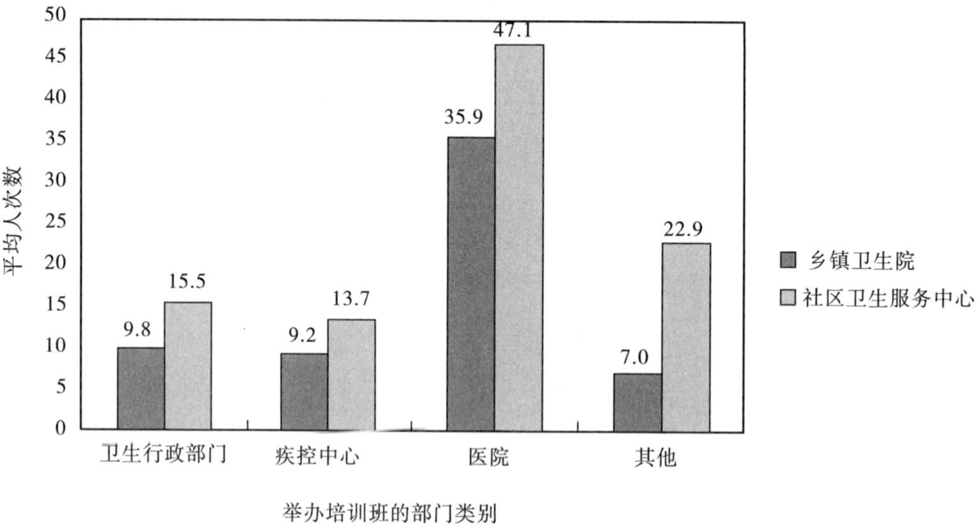

图 2-30 基层医疗卫生机构组织人员参加各类机构举办的慢性病防控相关培训班的平均人次数

3. 培训需求情况

2011 年，对各级疾控中心工作人员慢性病相关技能培训的需求情况做了调查。调查发现各级、各地疾控中心对 8 项技能培训的需求都较高，其中需求最高的比例为 92.6%，最低的为 86.9%（表 2-37、表 2-38）。

表 2-37 各级疾控中心慢性病防控相关培训技能需求情况 [机构数（%）]

级别	数据统计分析技能	死因监测技能	慢性病及危险因素监测技能	健康教育和健康促进技能	高危人群管理相关技能	患者管理相关技能	慢性病防控基础及综合技能	慢性病评估与报告撰写技能
省级	31（96.9）	25（78.1）	25（78.1）	28（87.5）	30（93.8）	26（81.3）	24（75.0）	27（84.4）
地市级	319（92.2）	312（90.2）	326（94.2）	305（88.2）	326（94.2）	321（92.8）	321（92.8）	325（93.9）
县（区）级	2610（88.9）	2545（86.7）	2642（90.0）	2587（88.1）	2712（92.3）	2681（91.3）	2669（90.9）	2645（90.1）
合计	**2960（89.3）**	**2882（86.9）**	**2993（90.3）**	**2920（88.1）**	**3068（92.6）**	**3028（91.3）**	**3014（90.9）**	**2997（90.4）**

表 2-38　各地疾控中心慢性病防控相关培训技能需求情况［机构数（%）］

地区	数据统计分析技能	死因监测技能	慢性病及危险因素监测技能	健康教育和健康促进技能	高危人群管理相关技能	患者管理相关技能	慢性病防控基础及综合技能	慢性病评估与报告撰写技能
东部	918（92.5）	860（86.5）	899（90.5）	861（86.7）	923（93.0）	897（90.3）	893（89.9）	911（91.7）
中部	882（88.6）	871（87.5）	911（91.6）	875（87.9）	922（92.7）	910（91.5）	905（91.0）	906（91.1）
西部	1160（87.4）	1151（86.7）	1183（89.2）	1184（89.2）	1223（92.2）	1221（92.0）	1216（91.6）	1180（88.9）
合计	2960（89.3）	2882（86.9）	2993（90.3）	2920（88.1）	3068（92.6）	3028（91.3）	3014（90.9）	2997（90.4）

（二）技术指导能力

慢性病防控现场工作（技术）指导，主要指各级疾控中心和基层医疗卫生机构对其技术指导单位开展慢性病防控相关工作（技术）指导的情况。具体包括，省级和地市级疾控中心对县（区）级疾控中心的指导；县（区）级疾控中心对基层医疗卫生机构的指导和基层医疗卫生机构对社区卫生服务站或村卫生室的指导。

2011 年，全国有 30 个省级疾控中心开展过对县（区）级疾控中心的现场指导工作，占机构比例为 93.8%（2009 年为 100%），85.5%的地市级疾控中心指导过县（区）级疾控中心（2009 年为 64.7%），东、中、西部地区呈现递减趋势。79.5%的县（区）级疾控中心开展过对基层医疗卫生机构的指导工作（2009 年为 48.3%），这一比例也呈现东、中、西部递减趋势（图 2-31）。

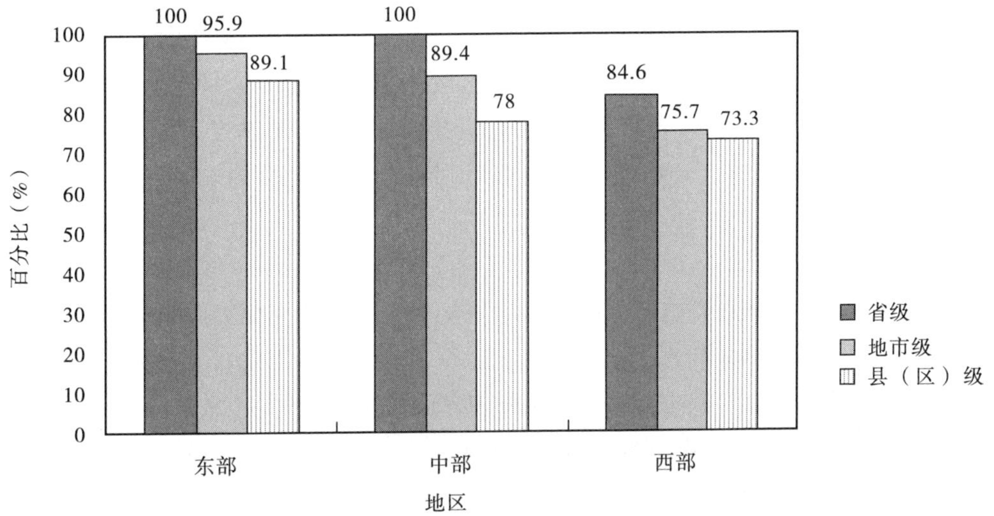

图 2-31　各地、各级疾控中心开展现场工作指导的比例

［省级、地市级指导县（区）级疾控中心/县（区）级疾控中心指导基层医疗卫生机构］

2011 年，省级疾控中心指导县（区）级疾控中心的平均次数为 3. 1 次，其中东部地区最高，平均次数为 3. 7 次。地市级疾控中心对县（区）级疾控中心的现场指导次数偏低，平均指导 2. 8 次。县（区）级疾控中心对基层医疗卫生机构开展指导的次数平均为 30. 0 次，其中东部地区最高，平均为 41. 4 次（图 2-32）。

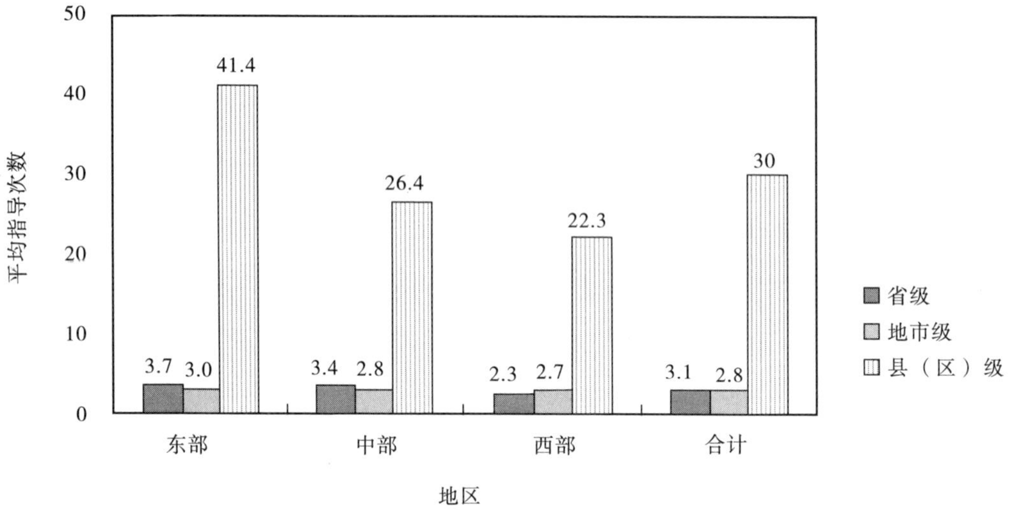

图 2-32　各地、各级疾控中心开展现场工作指导的平均次数

［省级、地市级指导县（区）级疾控中心/县（区）级疾控中心指导基层医疗卫生机构］

2011 年，全国有 2160 个基层医疗卫生机构对辖区内的社区卫生服务站/村卫生室开展慢性病现场技术指导，占被调查机构的比例为 73. 1%（2009 年为 49. 0%），其中乡镇卫生院 1220 个，比例为 82. 6%（2009 年为 36. 9%）、社区卫生服务中心 940 个，比例为 63. 6%（2009 年为 60. 8%）。从地区分布来看，开展现场技术指导工作的基层医疗卫生机构的比例东部最高，为 74. 5%，其次为中、西部，分别为 74. 1%、70. 7%。

（三）知识普及能力

知识普及能力主要指被调查基层医疗卫生机构在慢性病防控相关健康主题日（主要包括世界高血压日、世界糖尿病日、全民健康日、全民健康生活方式日、世界无烟日、世界脑卒中日和世界心脏病日等）期间开展相关知识宣传活动的情况。

2011 年，被调查基层医疗卫生机构在高血压日开展活动的比例最高，达 91. 0%，较 2009 年（56. 3%）有大幅度增加，其中社区卫生服务中心为 96. 5%、乡镇卫生院的比例为 85. 4%。在世界无烟日、世界糖尿病日、全民健康生活方式日、世界脑卒中日和世界心脏病日开展过相关宣传活动的机构比例依次降低，分别为 88. 5%、87. 8%、68. 2%、48. 5%和

41.8%（图 2-33）。

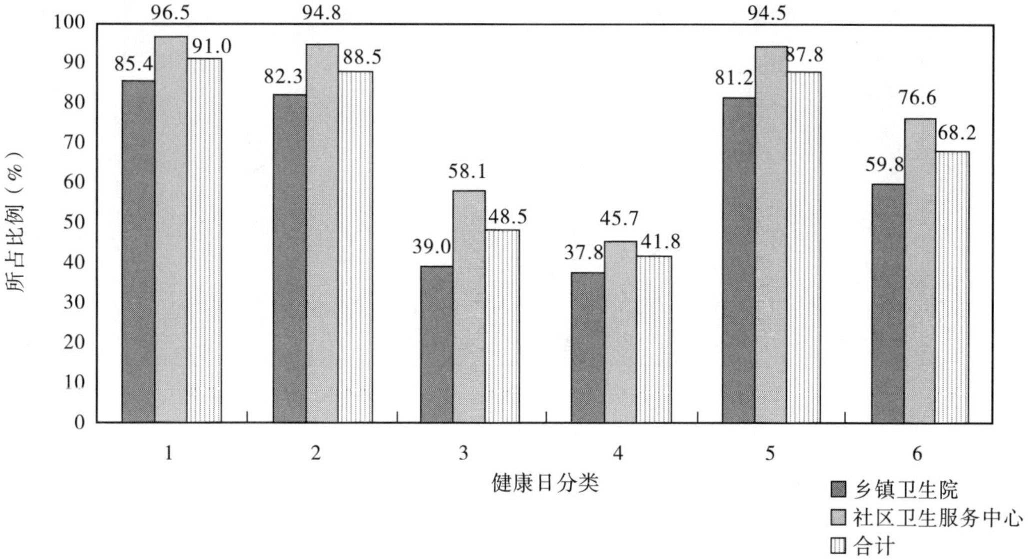

图 2-33　全国基层医疗卫生机构在慢性病防控相关健康日期间开展相关知识宣传活动的情况

分类（X）轴上，健康日分类，各数值所代表的含义：1. 高血压日宣传活动；2. 无烟日宣传活动；3. 脑卒中日宣传活动；4. 心脏病日宣传活动；5. 糖尿病日宣传活动；6. 全民健康生活方式日宣传活动

五、慢性病防控合作与参与能力

慢性病防控合作与参与能力是一个广义的概念，它包括与其他机构或部门在慢性病防控领域开展项目合作的能力和参与上级机构慢性病防控相关工作的能力。

（一）合作能力

2011 年，36.2%的疾控中心与媒体开展过合作，居首位，且高于 2009 年的 20.2%。与独立健康教育机构、专业防办、二级及以上医院和 NGO 等其他机构合作的比例分别为 13.6%、6.1%、28.2%和 5.9%。开展慢性病防控相关合作的各级疾控中心的比例由高到低依次为省级、地市级、县（区）级。其中，省级疾控中心与媒体或二级以上医院开展合作的机构比例分别均为 71.9%明显高于与其他机构合作的比例（图 2-34）。从地区分布来看，东部疾控中心与其他机构合作的比例高于中、西部地区（图 2-35）。

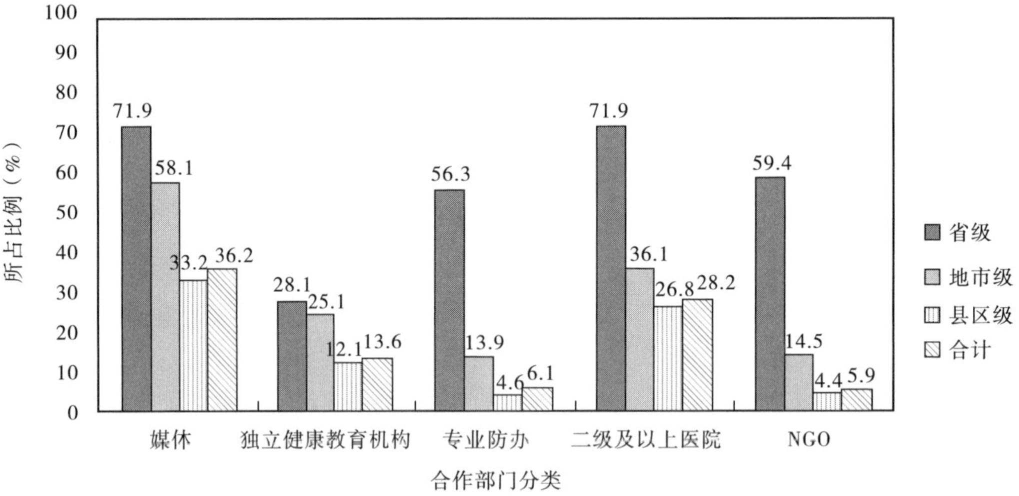

图 2-34　各级疾控中心开展慢性病防控相关合作情况

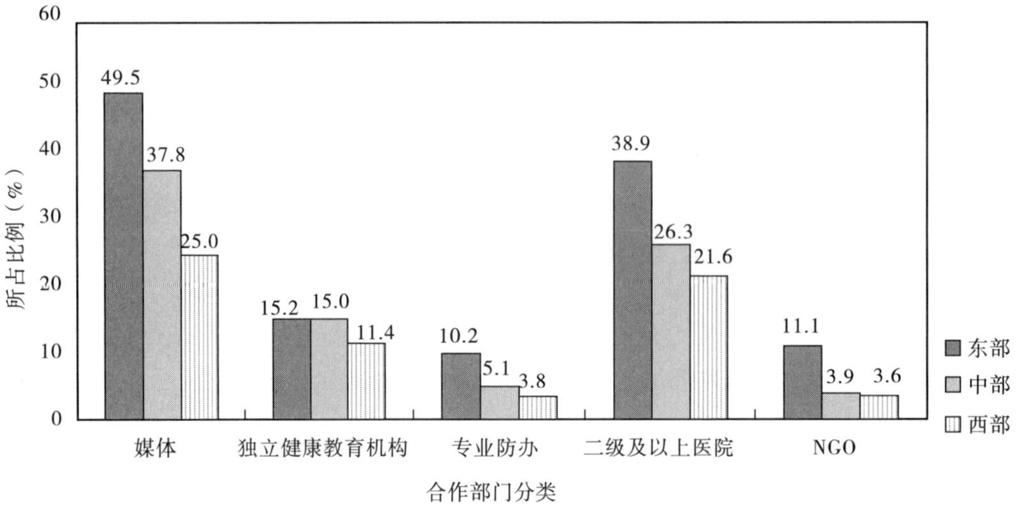

图 2-35　不同地区疾控中心开展慢性病防控相关合作情况

2011 年，各级教育部门、体育部门、环保部门、财政部门、农业部门等非卫生领域的机构参与慢性病防控工作的比例分别为 19.2%、10.1%、3.5%、11.4%和 2.8%。非卫生领域各部门参与慢性病防控工作的比例基本呈省、地市、县（区）和东、中、西递减趋势（图 2-36 和图 2-37）。

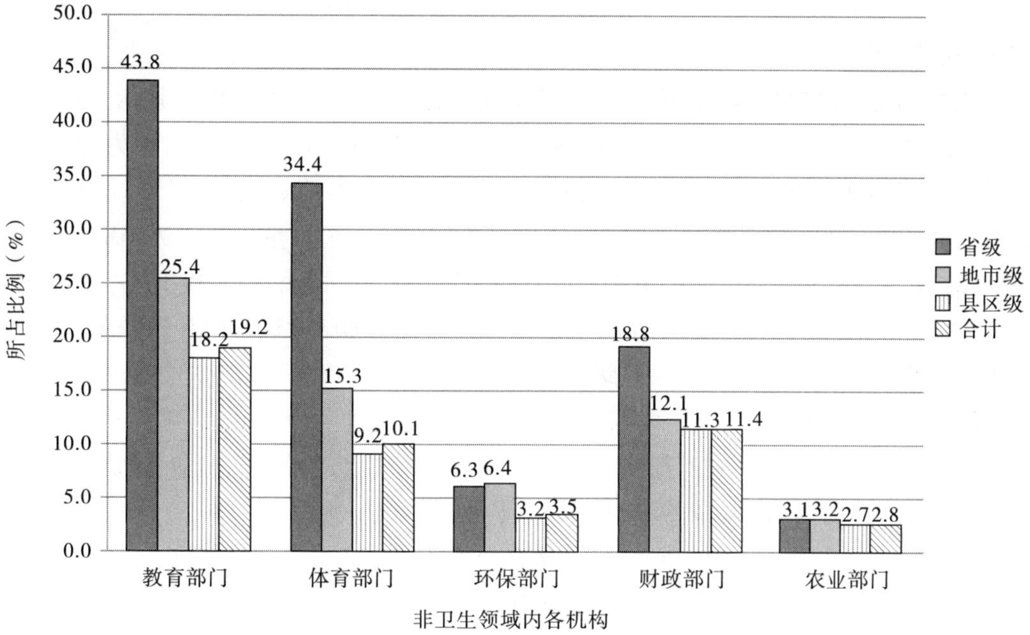

图 2-36　各级非卫生领域内各机构参与慢性病防控相关工作的情况

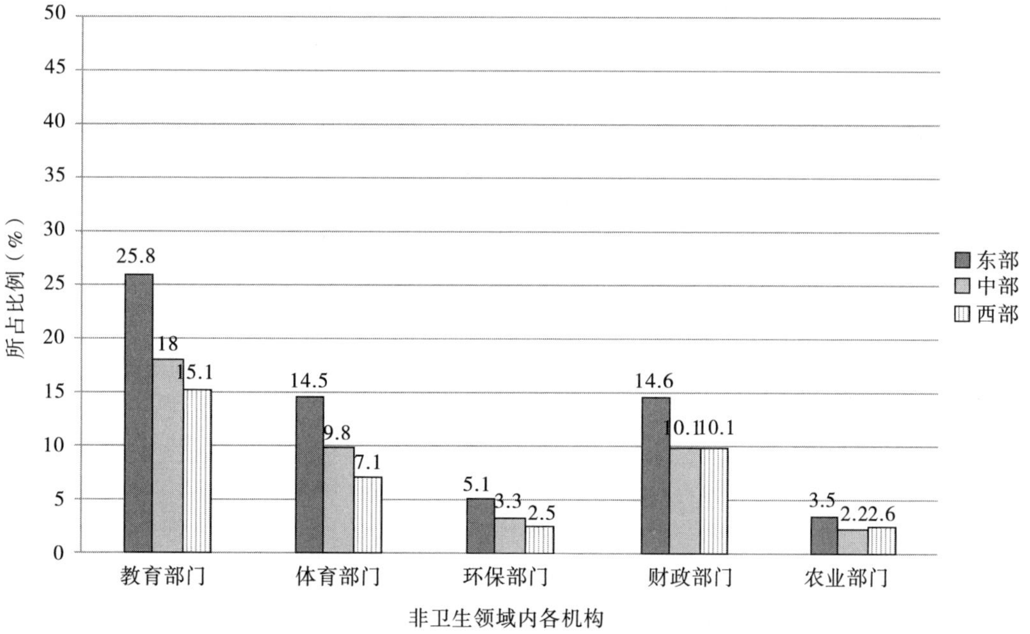

图 2-37　不同地区非卫生领域内各机构参与慢性病防控相关工作的情况

（二）参与能力

1. 疾控中心

参与能力主要以参与本级卫生行政部门政策制定、参与本级卫生以外其他行政部门慢性病防控工作和参与上级卫生行政部门或业务机构慢性病防控工作等三个方面为衡量。

参与本级卫生行政部门政策制定的各级疾控中心比例，省、地市、县（区）分别为59.4%、30.9%和29.1%；其中，地市级和县（区）级疾控中心参与的比例分别高于2009年的21.1%和14.3%，省级低于2009年的65.6%；东部地区（35.5%）高于中部（26.6%）和西部（27.4%）。参与本级卫生以外其他行政部门慢性病防控工作的各级疾控中心比例，省级、地市级、县（区）级分别为62.5%、34.4%和29.7%，分别高于2009年的省级46.9%、地市级19.4%和县（区）级12.4%；地区分布由高到低依次为东部（35.5%）、中部（29.6%）和西部（27.4%）。参与上级卫生行政部门或业务机构慢性病防控工作的各级疾控中心比例，省级、地市级、县（区）级分别为71.9%、28.6%和18.0%，高于2009年的68.8%、14.2%和8.1%，地区分布由高到低依次为东部（22.7%）、西部（18.7%）和中部（17.8%）（表2-39、表2-40和表2-41）。

表2-39 各地、各级疾控中心参与本级卫生行政部门政策制定的情况［机构数（%）］

级别	东部	中部	西部	合计
省级	9（81.8）	4（50.0）	6（46.2）	19（59.4）
地市级	45（45.9）	25（24.0）	37（25.7）	107（30.9）
县（区）级	298（33.7）	236（26.7）	320（27.4）	854（29.1）
合计	**352（35.5）**	**265（26.6）**	**363（27.4）**	**980（29.6）**

表2-40 各地、各级疾控中心参与本级卫生以外其他行政部门慢性病防控工作的情况［机构数（%）］

级别	东部	中部	西部	合计
省级	9（81.8）	6（75.0）	5（38.5）	20（62.5）
地市级	45（45.9）	34（32.7）	40（27.8）	119（34.4）
县（区）级	299（33.8）	254（28.8）	318（27.2）	871（29.7）
合计	**353（35.5）**	**294（29.6）**	**363（27.4）**	**1010（30.5）**

表 2-41　各地、各级疾控中心参与上级卫生行政部门或业务机构慢性病防控工作的情况［机构数（%）］

级别	东部	中部	西部	合计
省级	9（81.8）	7（87.5）	7（53.9）	23（71.9）
地市级	42（42.9）	20（19.2）	37（25.7）	99（28.6）
县（区）级	174（19.7）	150（17.0）	204（17.4）	528（18.0）
合计	**225（22.7）**	**177（17.8）**	**248（18.7）**	**650（19.6）**

2. 基层医疗卫生机构

被调查基层医疗卫生机构参与慢性病防控相关项目或科研工作的比例为 12.4%，其中乡镇卫生院为 7.1%，社区卫生服务中心为 17.7%。从地区分布来看，以东部地区的基层医疗卫生机构参与慢性病防控相关项目或科研工作的比例最高，为 15.9%，中部和西部分别为 12.0%和 8.8%。

被调查基层医疗卫生机构中参与国家级慢性病防控相关项目或科研工作的比例为 4.8%，其中社区卫生服务中心为 7.6%，乡镇卫生院为 2.0%；从地区分布来看，东部地区的参与的比例最高（6.6%），中、西部地区为 4.1%和 3.3%。

被调查基层医疗卫生机构中参与省级慢性病防控相关项目或科研工作的比例为 2.9%，其中社区卫生服务中心为 4.3%，乡镇卫生院仅为 1.5%；从地区分布来看，东部地区的参与的比例最高（4.5%），中、西部地区为 3.3%和 0.8%。

被调查基层医疗卫生机构中参与地市级慢性病防控相关项目或科研工作的比例为 3.2%，其中社区卫生服务中心为 5.5%，乡镇卫生院仅为 0.9%；从地区分布来看，东部地区的参与的比例最高（4.6%），中、西部地区分别为 3.1%和 1.7%。

被调查基层医疗卫生机构中参与县（区）级慢性病防控相关项目或科研工作的比例为 5.5%，其中社区卫生服务中心为 7.0%，乡镇卫生院为 4.1%；从地区分布来看，东部地区的参与的比例最高（6.6%），中、西部地区分别为 4.5%和 5.1%（图 2-38、图 2-39）。

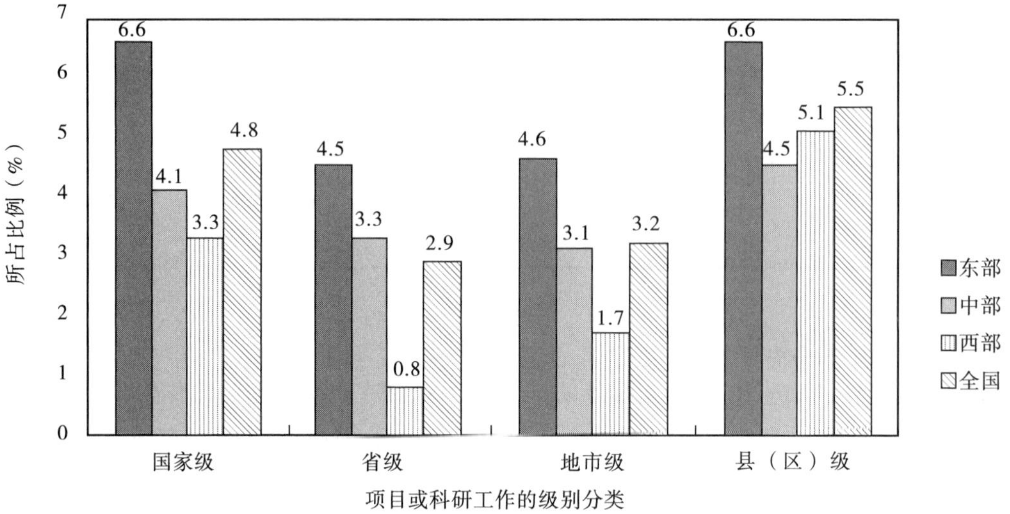

图 2-38　各地区基层医疗卫生机构参与各级慢性病防控相关项目或科研工作的情况

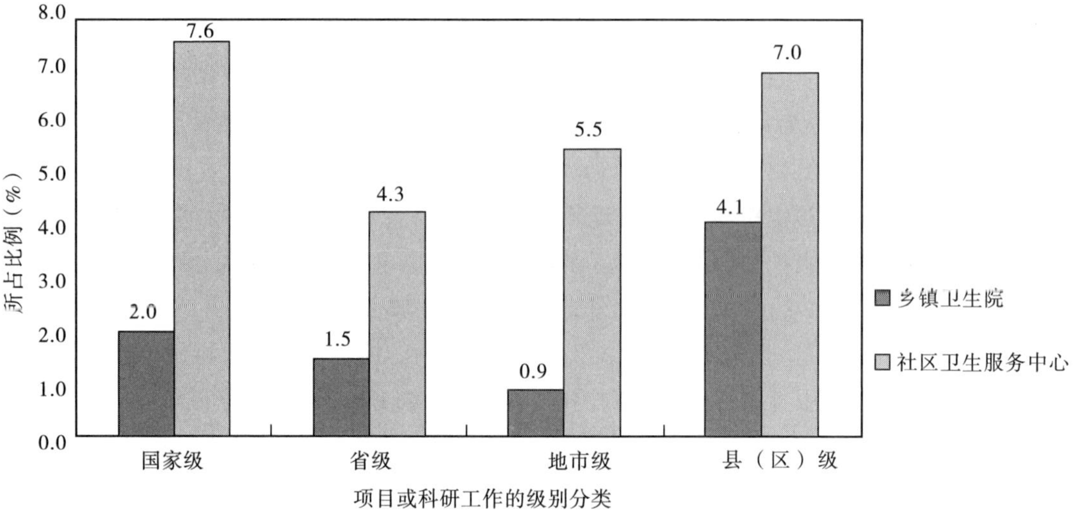

图 2-39　各类基层医疗卫生机构参与各级慢性病防控相关项目或科研工作的情况

六、慢性病监测能力

慢性病监测主要包括：死因监测、慢性病危险因素监测、慢性病发病和患病登记等。慢性病监测能力主要通过各级、各地慢性病监测工作的开展情况来反映。

（一）死因监测

1. 疾控中心

（1）开展情况

2011年全国有66.1%的疾控中心所在地区开展了死因监测工作，比例与2009年（66.3%）相当。省级、地市级、县（区）级开展此项工作的比例分别为96.9%、80.1%和63.4%，地市级开展死因监测的比例比2009年（77.7%）有所上升，省级和县（区）级比2009年（100%和64.6%）均有小幅度下降。从地区分布来看，开展死因监测工作的比例呈东、中、西下降趋势，与2009年的分布情况一致（表2-42）。

表2-42　各地、各级疾控中心所在地开展死因监测工作情况［机构数（%）］

级别	东部	中部	西部	合计
省级	11（100.0）	8（100.0）	12（92.3）	31（96.9）
地市级	92（93.9）	84（80.8）	101（70.1）	277（80.1）
县（区）级	713（80.7）	578（65.5）	593（50.7）	1884（63.4）
合计	**816（82.2）**	**670（67.3）**	**706（53.2）**	**2192（66.1）**

（2）任务来源

在开展的死因监测工作中任务来源主要是上级，占93.3%，任务来源于本级的比例为32.4%，任务来源于国际的比例很低，仅为2.5%。省级、地市级和县（区）级死因监测任务来源于上级的比例分别为93.5%、92.1%、93.5%，从地区分布看，东部地区任务来源于上级的比例高于中、西部地区（表2-43、表2-44）。

表2-43　各级开展的死因监测工作中任务来源情况［机构数（%）］

地区	任务来源		
	国际	上级机构	本级机构
省级	0（0.0）	29（93.5）	15（48.4）
地市级	6（2.2）	255（92.1）	90（32.5）
县（区）级	48（2.5）	1761（93.5）	605（32.1）
合计	**54（2.5）**	**2045（93.3）**	**710（32.4）**

表 2-44　各地开展的死因监测工作中任务来源情况［机构数（%）］

地区	任务来源		
	国际	上级机构	本级机构
东部	8（1.0）	776（95.1）	262（32.1）
中部	20（2.5）	624（93.1）	193（28.8）
西部	26（3.2）	645（91.4）	255（36.1）
合计	**54（2.5）**	**2045（93.3）**	**710（32.4）**

（3）死因监测当地代表性情况

在开展死因监测的地区中，开展覆盖所有区县死因监测的省级比例为 48.4%，比例由高到低依次是东部地区、西部地区、中部地区，开展死因监测覆盖所有区县的地市级比例为 79.4%，地区分布上差异不大。开展死因监测工作覆盖所有街道和乡镇的县（区）级比例为 84.3%，东部地区最高，其次是西部（表 2-45）。

表 2-45　各地、各级疾控中心所在地开展覆盖所有区县/街道和乡镇的死因监测的比例［机构数（%）］

级别	东部	中部	西部	合计
省级	8（72.7）	2（25.0）	5（41.7）	15（48.4）
地市级	74（80.4）	66（78.6）	80（79.2）	220（79.4）
县（区）级	640（89.8）	457（79.1）	491（82.8）	1588（84.3）
合计	**722（88.5）**	**525（78.4）**	**576（81.6）**	**1823（83.2）**

各地、各级开展死因监测工作有当地代表性的比例为 6.8%，其中，省级、地市级、县（区）级疾控中心开展具有当地代表性的死因监测的比例分别为 22.6%、13.7%、5.5%，从地区分布来看，开展具有当地代表性的死因监测的比例东部地区低于中部与西部地区（表 2-46）。

表 2-46　各地、各级疾控中心所在地开展死因监测工作具有当地代表性的比例［机构数（%）］

级别	东部	中部	西部	合计
省级	2（18.2）	3（37.5）	2（16.7）	7（22.6）
地市级	12（13.0）	15（17.9）	11（10.9）	38（13.7）
县（区）级	33（4.6）	38（6.6）	33（5.6）	104（5.5）
合计	**47（5.8）**	**56（8.4）**	**46（6.5）**	**149（6.8）**

(4) 数据信息发布或利用情况

编写年报为死因监测数据发布或利用的首要形式，占59.0%，省级、地市级与县（区）级以编写年报发布或利用死因监测数据的比例分别为90.3%、64.3%、57.7%，2009年三级比例分别为84.4%、69.5%、56.8%。从地区分布来看，以编写年报形式发布或利用死因监测数据的比例从高到低依次是东部地区、中部地区、西部地区。省级以发表论文的形式发布或利用死因监测数据的比例（67.7%）高于地市级（23.1%）与县（区）级（7.3%），各级以发表论文的形式发布或利用死因监测数据的比例均高于2009年［省、地市、县（区）分别为56.3%、18.2%、5.8%］，从地区分布来看，以发表论文的形式发布或利用死因监测数据的比例东部地区高于中西部地区。以出版报告或媒体发布的形式发布或利用死因监测数据的比例均较低，分别为14.5%与3.4%，与2009年差别不大（图2-40、图2-41）。

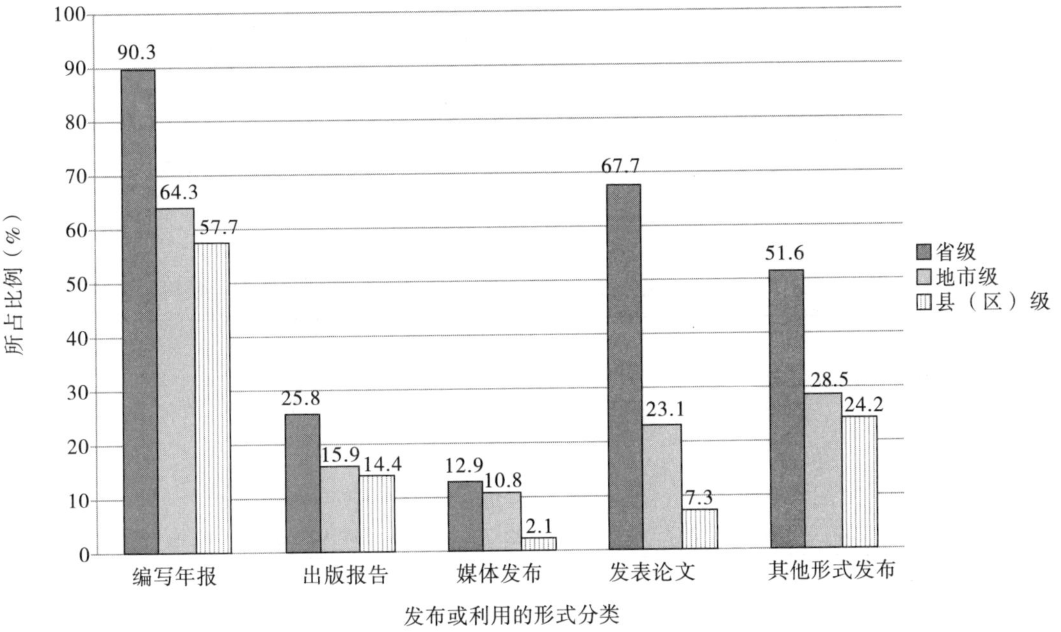

图2-40 各级疾控中心所在地区开展死因监测的数据信息发布或利用情况

各地、各级疾控中心所在地开展死因监测中信息被采纳的比例为54.8%，省级开展的死因监测信息被采纳率最高，为80.6%，其次是地市级62.8%，县（区）级最低，53.2%。从地区分布来看，西部地区开展的死因监测信息被采纳的比例略高于东部地区与中部地区（表2-47）。

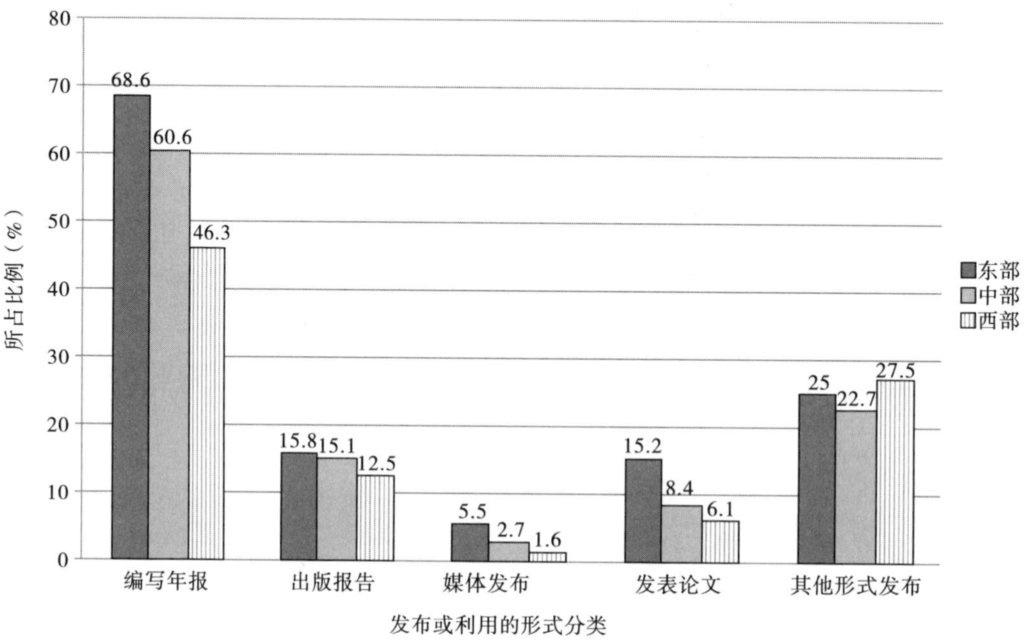

图 2-41 各地疾控中心所在地开展死因监测的数据信息发布或利用情况

表 2-47 各地、各级疾控中心所在地开展的死因监测中信息被采纳的比例［机构数（%）］

级别	东部	中部	西部	合计
省级	6（54.5）	5（62.5）	5（41.7）	25（80.6）
地市级	30（32.6）	16（19.0）	33（32.7）	174（62.8）
县（区）级	168（23.6）	131（22.7）	156（26.3）	1002（53.2）
合计	**204（25.0）**	**152（22.7）**	**194（27.5）**	**1201（54.8）**

2. 基层医疗卫生机构开展死亡病例报告情况

被调查基层医疗卫生机构开展死亡病例报告的比例为57.6%，比2009年（44.8%）有所上升，其中社区卫生服务中心开展死亡病例报告的比例为68.1%，高于2009年（56.6%），乡镇卫生院开展死亡病例报告的比例为47.2%，高于2009年（32.5%），从地区分布看，东部地区基层医疗卫生机构开展死亡病例报告的比例（74.2%）高于中西部地区（51.3%、44.0%）（表2-48）。

表 2-48　各地基层医疗卫生机构开展死亡病例报告情况［机构数（%）］

机构分类	东部	中部	西部	合计
乡镇卫生院	241（64.8）	215（46.0）	241（37.8）	697（47.2）
社区卫生服务中心	607（78.7）	194（58.6）	205（54.5）	1006（68.1）
合计	848（74.2）	409（51.3）	446（44.0）	1703（57.6）

（二）慢性病危险因素监测

1. 开展情况

慢性病相关危险因素主要包括烟草使用、膳食、身体活动、酒精使用、超重肥胖、血压、血糖和血脂等。从监测或调查的危险因素种类来看，2011 年，除血脂监测外，省级疾控中心所在地区开展各类慢性病危险因素监测的比例均在 90%以上，开展血糖与血脂监测的比例高于 2009 年，省级疾控中心所在地区开展各类危险因素监测的比例均高于地市级，地市级疾控中心所在地区开展各类危险因素监测的比例高于县（区）级，与 2009 年的情况一致。从地区分布来看，东部地区开展各类危险因素监测的比例高于中部和西部地区（表 2-50、表 2-49）。

表 2-49　各级疾控中心所在地开展慢性病相关危险因素监测或调查的情况［机构数（%）］

级别	烟草	膳食	身体活动	酒精使用	超重肥胖	血压	血糖	血脂
省级	30（93.8）	29（90.6）	30（93.8）	29（90.6）	30（93.8）	31（96.9）	31（96.9）	28（87.5）
地市级	165（47.7）	127（36.7）	123（35.5）	120（34.7）	127（36.7）	157（45.4）	148（42.8）	115（33.2）
县（区）级	795（27.1）	687（23.4）	655（22.3）	650（22.1）	683（23.3）	1043（35.5）	980（33.4）	577（19.6）
合计	990（29.9）	843（25.4）	808（24.4）	799（24.1）	840（25.3）	1231（37.1）	1159（35.0）	720（21.7）

表 2-50　不同地区疾控中心所在地开展慢性病相关危险因素监测或调查的情况［机构数（%）］

地区	烟草	膳食	身体活动	酒精使用	超重肥胖	血压	血糖	血脂
东部	438（44.1）	394（39.7）	381（38.4）	386（38.9）	394（39.7）	513（51.7）	484（48.7）	323（32.5）
中部	272（27.3）	221（22.2）	211（21.2）	198（19.9）	215（21.6）	329（33.1）	307（30.9）	194（19.5）
西部	280（21.1）	228（17.2）	216（16.3）	215（16.2）	231（17.4）	389（29.3）	368（27.7）	203（15.3）
合计	990（29.9）	843（25.4）	808（24.4）	799（24.1）	840（25.3）	1231（37.1）	1159（35.0）	720（21.7）

2. 任务来源情况

2011 年不同地区、各级疾控中心所在地开展烟草使用、膳食、身体活动、酒精使用、超重肥胖、血压、血糖和血脂的调查工作任务中主要来源为上级机构的比例最高，其次是本级（图 2-42）。

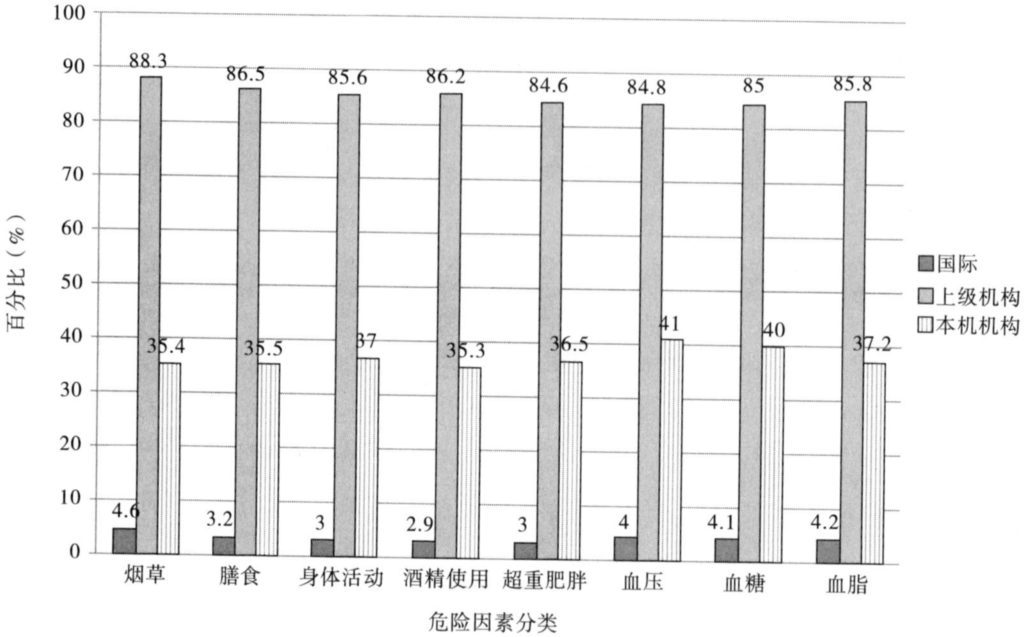

图 2-42　2011 年各类慢性病危险因素监测工作任务来源情况

3. 覆盖所有县区/乡镇和街道的情况

省级开展烟草调查覆盖所有县（区）的比例为 16.7%，其中东部最高，为 27.3%，其次是西部。地市级开展烟草调查覆盖所有县（区）的比例为 38.2%，东部略低于中、西部地区。县（区）级开展烟草调查覆盖所有乡镇和街道的比例为 59.0%，西部地区最高（64.9%）（表 2-51）。

表 2-51　各地、各级疾控中心所在地开展覆盖所有县（区）/街道和乡镇的烟草调查的比例 [机构数（%）]

级别	东部	中部	西部	合计
省级	3（27.3）	0（0.0）	2（18.2）	5（16.7）
地市级	25（37.9）	20（38.5）	18（38.3）	63（38.2）

续　表

级别	东部	中部	西部	合计
县（区）级	193（53.5）	132（62.3）	144（64.9）	469（59.0）
合计	**221（50.5）**	**152（55.9）**	**164（58.6）**	**537（54.2）**

省级开展膳食调查覆盖所有县（区）的比例为13.8%。地市级开展膳食调查覆盖所有县（区）的比例为36.2%，其中中部地区开展膳食调查覆盖所有县（区）的比例最高为43.6%，最低为西部地区（30.3%）。县（区）级开展膳食调查覆盖所有乡镇和街道的比例为56.8%，其中西部地区最高（63.6%）（表2-52）。

表2-52　各地、各级疾控中心所在地开展覆盖所有县（区）/街道和乡镇的膳食调查的比例［机构数（%）］

级别	东部	中部	西部	合计
省级	2（18.2）	0（0.0）	2（18.2）	4（13.8）
地市级	19（34.5）	17（43.6）	10（30.3）	46（36.2）
县（区）级	176（53.7）	97（55.4）	117（63.6）	390（56.8）
合计	**197（50.0）**	**114（51.6）**	**129（56.6）**	**440（52.2）**

省级开展身体活动调查覆盖所有县（区）的比例为13.3%。地市级开展身体活动调查覆盖所有县（区）的比例为35.0%，其中中部地区最高（43.6%），西部地区最低（28.1%）。县（区）级开展身体活动调查覆盖所有乡镇和街道的比例为57.4%，其中西部地区最高（64.0%）（表2-53）。

表2-53　各地、各级疾控中心所在地开展覆盖所有县（区）/街道和乡镇的身体活动调查的比例［机构数（%）］

级别	东部	中部	西部	合计
省级	2（18.2）	0（0.0）	2（16.7）	4（13.3）
地市级	17（32.7）	17（43.6）	9（28.1）	43（35.0）
县（区）级	170（53.5）	96（58.2）	110（64.0）	376（57.4）
合计	**189（49.6）**	**113（53.6）**	**121（56.0）**	**423（52.4）**

省级开展酒精使用调查覆盖所有县（区）的比例为 13.8%。地市级开展酒精使用调查覆盖所有县（区）的比例为 35.8%，其中中部地区比例最高为 44.7%，西部地区比例最低为 27.6%。县（区）级开展酒精使用调查覆盖所有乡镇和街道的比例为 58.0%，其中西部地区最高为 65.1%（表 2-54）。

表 2-54 各地、各级疾控中心所在地开展覆盖所有县（区）/街道和乡镇的酒精使用调查的比例［机构数（%）］

级别	东部	中部	西部	合计
省级	2（18.2）	0（0.0）	2（18.2）	4（13.8）
地市级	18（34.0）	17（44.7）	8（27.6）	43（35.8）
县（区）级	174（54.0）	89（58.2）	114（65.1）	377（58.0）
合计	**194（50.3）**	**105（53.0）**	**124（57.7）**	**424（53.1）**

省级开展超重肥胖调查覆盖所有县（区）的比例为 13.3%。地市级开展超重肥胖调查覆盖所有县（区）的比例为 35.4%。县（区）级开展超重肥胖调查覆盖所有乡镇和街道的比例为 59.2%，其中西部地区最高为 67.4%（表 2-55）。

表 2-55 各地、各级疾控中心所在地开展覆盖所有县（区）/街道和乡镇的超重或肥胖调查的比例［机构数（%）］

级别	东部	中部	西部	合计
省级	2（18.2）	0（0.0）	2（16.7）	4（13.3）
地市级	19（34.5）	17（40.5）	9（30.0）	45（35.4）
县（区）级	177（54.0）	99（59.6）	128（67.7）	404（59.2）
合计	**198（50.3）**	**116（54.0）**	**139（60.2）**	**453（53.9）**

省级开展血压调查覆盖所有县（区）的比例为 16.1%，其中东部最高为 18.2%。地市级开展血压调查覆盖所有县（区）的比例为 43.3%，其中西部地区比例最高为 48.9%，东部地区比例最低为 39.7%。县（区）级疾控中心开展血压调查覆盖所有乡镇和街道的比例为 71.7%，其中西部地区最高为 77.6%（表 2-56）。

表 2-56　各地、各级疾控中心所在地开展覆盖所有县（区）/街道和乡镇的血压调查的比例［机构数（%）］

级别	东部	中部	西部	合计
省级	2（18.2）	0（0.0）	2（16.7）	5（16.1）
地市级	25（39.7）	20（42.6）	23（48.9）	68（43.3）
县（区）级	291（66.3）	201（73.4）	256（77.6）	748（71.7）
合计	**318（62.0）**	**222（67.5）**	**282（72.5）**	**821（66.7）**

省级开展血糖调查覆盖所有县（区）的比例为9.7%，其中西部最高为16.7%。地市级开展血糖调查覆盖所有县（区）的比例为44.6%，其中西部地区比例最高为48.9%。县（区）级开展血糖调查覆盖所有乡镇和街道的比例为71.8%，其中西部地区最高为77.8%（表2-57）。

表 2-57　各地、各级疾控中心所在地开展覆盖所有县（区）/街道和乡镇的血糖调查的比例［机构数（%）］

级别	东部	中部	西部	合计
省级	1（9.1）	0（0.0）	2（16.7）	3（9.7）
地市级	25（42.4）	19（43.2）	22（48.9）	66（44.6）
县（区）级	271（65.5）	191（74.9）	242（77.8）	704（71.8）
合计	**297（61.4）**	**210（68.4）**	**266（72.3）**	**773（66.7）**

省级开展血脂调查覆盖所有县（区）的比例为7.1%。地市级开展血脂调查覆盖所有县（区）的比例为38.3%。县（区）级开展血脂调查覆盖所有乡镇和街道的比例为58.9%（表2-58）。

表 2-58　各地、各级疾控中心所在地开展覆盖所有县（区）/街道和乡镇的血脂调查的比例［机构数（%）］

级别	东部	中部	西部	合计
省级	1（9.1）	0（0.0）	1（10.0）	2（7.1）
地市级	14（30.4）	16（44.4）	14（42.4）	44（38.3）
县（区）级	139（52.3）	98（64.9）	103（64.4）	340（58.9）
合计	**154（47.7）**	**114（58.8）**	**118（58.1）**	**386（53.6）**

4. 具有当地代表性的情况

在各地开展的各类危险因素监测中，有的虽没有覆盖本地区所有县（区）或乡镇但其样本量具有当地代表性。其中烟草使用、膳食、身体活动、酒精使用、超重肥胖、血压、血糖和血脂监测具有当地代表性的比例等分别为 34.3%、36.3%、35.3%、27.5%、34.0%、24.1%、23.4%、33.3%（表 2-59、表 2-60）。

表 2-59　各级疾控中心所在地开展的慢性病相关危险因素监测或调查中具有当地代表性情况［机构数（%）］

级别	烟草	膳食	身体活动	酒精使用	超重肥胖	血压	血糖	血脂
省级	14（46.7）	14（48.3）	13（43.3）	0（0.0）	15（50.0）	14（45.2）	13（41.9）	13（46.4）
地市级	64（38.8）	48（37.8）	47（38.2）	0（0.0）	48（37.8）	52（33.1）	47（31.8）	42（36.5）
县（区）级	262（33.0）	244（35.5）	225（34.4）	220（33.8）	223（32.7）	231（22.1）	211（21.5）	185（32.1）
合计	**340（34.3）**	**306（36.3）**	**285（35.3）**	**220（27.5）**	**286（34.0）**	**297（24.1）**	**271（23.4）**	**240（33.3）**

表 2-60　不同地区疾控中心所在地开展的慢性病相关危险因素监测或调查中具有当地代表性情况［机构数（%）］

地区	烟草	膳食	身体活动	酒精使用	超重肥胖	血压	血糖	血脂
东部	174（39.7）	158（40.1）	150（39.4）	121（31.3）	155（39.3）	154（30.0）	143（29.5）	129（39.9）
中部	91（33.5）	78（35.3）	68（32.2）	48（24.2）	67（31.2）	68（20.7）	61（19.9）	57（29.4）
西部	75（26.8）	70（30.7）	67（31.0）	51（23.7）	64（27.7）	75（19.3）	67（18.2）	54（26.6）
合计	**340（34.3）**	**306（36.3）**	**285（35.3）**	**220（27.5）**	**286（34.0）**	**297（24.1）**	**271（23.4）**	**240（33.3）**

5. 信息发布或利用情况

在各地、各级疾控中心所在地开展的各类慢性病危险因素监测中，编写年报均是其数据信息发布及利用的首要形式，之后依次为其他形式和发表论文，以出版报告或媒体发布的形式发布及利用慢性病危险因素监测数据的比例在各级均较低，与 2009 年调查结果一致（图 2-43）。

6. 信息被采纳的情况

2011 年各地、各级疾控中心所在地开展各类慢性病危险因素监测信息被采纳的比例较低，烟草使用、膳食、身体活动、酒精使用、超重肥胖、血压、血糖、血脂等信息被采纳的比例分别为 65.5%、67.9%、68.6%、67.8%、67.1%、62.9%、63.7%、65.1%。从地区分布来看，各类慢性病危险因素监测中信息被采纳的比例东部地区均高于中、西部地区（表 2-61、表 2-62）。

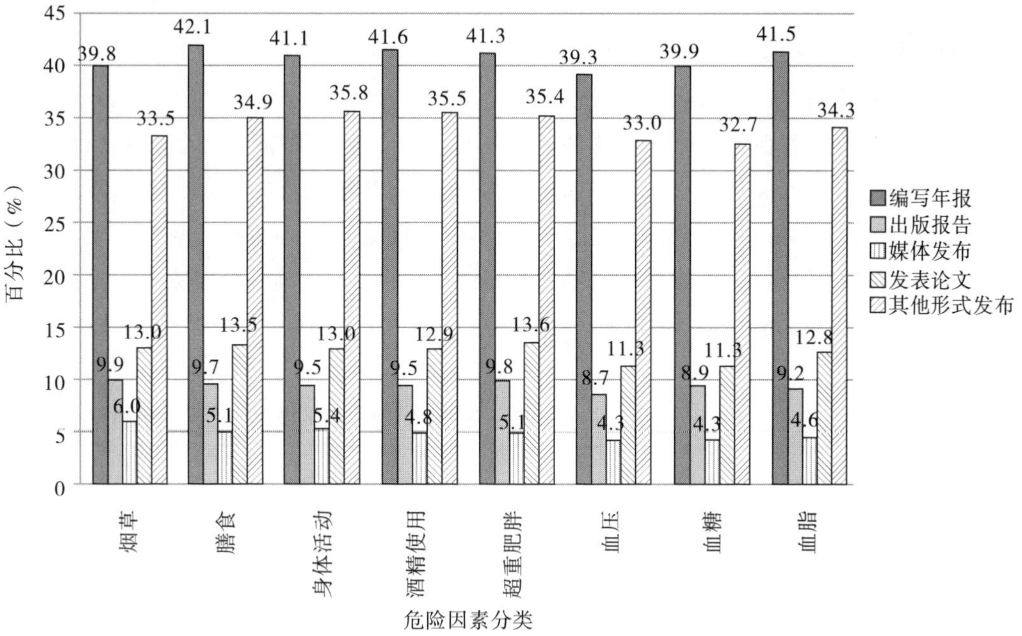

图 2-43　各类慢性病危险因素监测数据信息发布及利用情况

表 2-61　各级疾控中心所在地开展慢性病相关危险因素监测或调查中信息被采纳的情况［机构数（%）］

级别	烟草	膳食	身体活动	酒精使用	超重肥胖	血压	血糖	血脂
省级	19（63.3）	18（62.1）	18（60.0）	17（58.6）	19（63.3）	20（64.5）	19（61.3）	18（64.3）
地市级	108（65.5）	83（65.4）	78（63.4）	75（62.5）	77（60.6）	100（63.7）	95（64.2）	71（61.7）
县（区）级	521（65.5）	471（68.6）	458（70.0）	450（69.3）	468（68.5）	654（62.7）	624（63.7）	380（65.9）
合计	**648（65.5）**	**572（67.9）**	**554（68.6）**	**542（67.8）**	**564（67.1）**	**774（62.9）**	**738（63.7）**	**469（65.1）**

表 2-62　不同地区疾控中心所在地开展慢性病相关危险因素监测或调查中信息被采纳的情况［机构数（%）］

地区	烟草	膳食	身体活动	酒精使用	超重肥胖	血压	血糖	血脂
东部	314（71.7）	290（73.6）	283（74.3）	283（73.3）	291（73.9）	360（70.2）	345（71.3）	235（72.8）
中部	152（55.9）	122（55.2）	120（56.9）	111（56.1）	122（56.7）	181（55.0）	172（56.0）	108（55.7）
西部	182（65.0）	160（70.2）	151（69.9）	148（68.8）	151（65.4）	233（59.9）	221（60.1）	126（62.1）
合计	**648（65.5）**	**572（67.9）**	**554（68.6）**	**542（67.8）**	**564（67.1）**	**774（62.9）**	**738（63.7）**	**469（65.1）**

(三) 发病和患病登记/报告

1. 疾控中心

(1) 发病和患病登记/报告开展情况

各地、各级疾控中心所在地开展恶性肿瘤病例报告、脑卒中病例报告、心肌梗死病例报告的比例分别为 35.5%、22.3%和 21.1%，均高于 2009 年调查的结果（29.2%、19.0%、17.6%），其中省级开展恶性肿瘤病例报告、脑卒中病例报告、心肌梗死病例报告的比例均高于地市级与县（区）级，与 2009 年调查的分布情况一致。从地区分布来看，东部地区高于中、西部地区（表 2-63、表 2-64）。

表 2-63 各级疾控中心所在地开展恶性肿瘤、脑卒中和心肌梗死病例报告的情况［机构数（%）］

级别	恶性肿瘤	脑卒中	心肌梗死
省级	29（90.6）	13（40.6）	12（37.5）
地市级	168（48.6）	87（25.1）	83（24.0）
县（区）级	981（33.4）	638（21.7）	605（20.6）
合计	**1178（35.5）**	**738（22.3）**	**700（21.1）**

表 2-64 不同地区疾控中心所在地开展恶性肿瘤、脑卒中和心肌梗死病例报告的情况［机构数（%）］

地区	恶性肿瘤	脑卒中	心肌梗死
东部	570（57.4）	358（36.1）	342（34.4）
中部	292（29.3）	175（17.6）	170（17.1）
西部	316（23.8）	205（15.4）	188（14.2）
合计	**1178（35.5）**	**738（22.3）**	**700（21.1）**

(2) 发病和患病登记/报告任务来源情况

各地、各级开展恶性肿瘤病例报告、脑卒中病例报告、心肌梗死病例报告工作任务来源均以上级机构为主，分别为 91.5%、84.4%、83.9%；从地区分布来看，各地开展恶性肿瘤病例报告、脑卒中病例报告、心肌梗死病例报告工作任务来源均以上级机构为主（表 2-65、表 2-66、表 2-67、表 2-68、表 2-69、表 2-70）。

表 2-65　各级疾控中心所在地开展恶性肿瘤报告工作任务来源情况［机构数（%）］

级别	任务来源		
	国际	上级机构	本级机构
省级	0（0.0）	23（79.3）	13（44.8）
地市级	4（2.4）	148（88.1）	60（35.7）
县（区）级	20（2.0）	907（92.5）	325（33.1）
合计	**24（2.0）**	**1078（91.5）**	**398（33.8）**

表 2-66　不同地区疾控中心所在地开展恶性肿瘤报告工作任务来源情况［机构数（%）］

级别	任务来源		
	国际	上级机构	本级机构
东部	6（1.1）	540（94.7）	182（31.9）
中部	8（2.7）	255（87.3）	92（31.5）
西部	10（3.2）	283（89.6）	124（39.2）
合计	**24（2.0）**	**1078（91.5）**	**398（33.8）**

表 2-67　各级疾控中心所在地开展脑卒中病例报告工作任务来源情况［机构数（%）］

级别	任务来源		
	国际	上级机构	本级机构
省级	0（0.0）	4（30.8）	9（69.2）
地市级	1（1.1）	57（65.5）	44（50.6）
县（区）级	13（2.0）	562（88.1）	249（39.0）
合计	**14（1.9）**	**623（84.4）**	**302（40.9）**

表 2-68　不同地区疾控中心所在地开展脑卒中病例报告工作任务来源情况［机构数（%）］

级别	任务来源		
	国际	上级机构	本级机构
东部	2（0.6）	313（87.4）	134（37.4）
中部	7（4.0）	137（78.3）	71（40.6）
西部	5（2.4）	173（84.4）	97（47.3）
合计	**14（1.9）**	**623（84.4）**	**302（40.9）**

表 2-69 各级疾控中心所在地开展心肌梗死病例报告工作任务来源情况 [机构数（%）]

级别	任务来源		
	国际	上级机构	本级机构
省级	0（0.0）	3（25.0）	9（75.0）
地市级	0（0.0）	54（65.1）	43（51.8）
县（区）级	11（1.8）	530（87.6）	239（39.5）
合计	**11（1.6）**	**587（83.9）**	**291（41.6）**

表 2-70 不同地区疾控中心所在地开展心肌梗死病例报告工作任务来源情况 [机构数（%）]

级别	任务来源		
	国际	上级机构	本级机构
东部	2（0.6）	300（87.7）	128（37.4）
中部	6（3.5）	133（78.2）	70（41.2）
西部	3（1.6）	154（81.9）	93（49.5）
合计	**11（1.6）**	**587（83.9）**	**291（41.6）**

（3）发病和患病登记/报告覆盖所有县区/街道和乡镇的情况

各级疾控中心开展覆盖所有县（区）/街道和乡镇的恶性肿瘤、脑卒中与心肌梗死病例报告的比例分别为 82.2%、86.3%、87.7%，县（区）级疾控中心开展覆盖所有街道和乡镇的恶性肿瘤、脑卒中与心肌梗死病例报告的比例分别为 89.2%、90.9%、92.1%。从地区分布看，开展覆盖所有县（区）/街道和乡镇的恶性肿瘤、脑卒中与心肌梗死病例报告的比例东部地区高于中、西部地区（表 2-71、表 2-72）。

表 2-71 各级疾控中心所在地开展恶性肿瘤、脑卒中和心肌梗死病例报告覆盖所有县（区）/街道和乡镇的情况 [机构数（%）]

级别	恶性肿瘤	脑卒中	心肌梗死
省级	6（20.7）	3（23.1）	3（25.0）
地市级	87（51.8）	54（62.1）	54（65.1）
县（区）级	875（89.2）	580（90.9）	557（92.1）
合计	**968（82.2）**	**637（86.3）**	**614（87.7）**

表 2-72　不同地区疾控中心所在地开展恶性肿瘤、脑卒中和心肌梗死病例报告覆盖所有县（区）/街道和乡镇的情况［机构数（%）］

地区	恶性肿瘤	脑卒中	心肌梗死
东部	489（85.8）	318（88.8）	308（90.1）
中部	244（83.6）	152（86.9）	149（87.6）
西部	235（74.4）	167（81.5）	157（83.5）
合计	**968（82.2）**	**637（86.3）**	**614（87.7）**

（4）发病和患病登记/报告具有当地代表性情况

在开展恶性肿瘤、脑卒中和心肌梗死病例的地区中，部分地区虽没有覆盖所有县（区）/街道和乡镇，但病例报告具有当地代表性。恶性肿瘤、脑卒中、心肌梗死病例报告的比例分别为9.7%、7.2%、6.3%（表2-73、表2-74）。

表 2-73　各级疾控中心所在地开展具有当地代表性的恶性肿瘤、脑卒中和心肌梗死病例报告的情况［机构数（%）］

级别	恶性肿瘤	脑卒中	心肌梗死
省级	9（31.0）	2（15.4）	2（16.7）
地市级	53（31.5）	16（18.4）	15（18.1）
县（区）级	52（5.3）	35（5.5）	27（4.5）
合计	**114（9.7）**	**53（7.2）**	**44（6.3）**

表 2-74　不同地区疾控中心所在地开展具有当地代表性的恶性肿瘤、脑卒中和心肌梗死病例报告的情况［机构数（%）］

地区	恶性肿瘤	脑卒中	心肌梗死
东部	39（6.8）	24（6.7）	20（5.8）
中部	29（9.9）	8（4.6）	8（4.7）
西部	46（14.6）	21（10.2）	16（8.5）
合计	**114（9.7）**	**53（7.2）**	**44（6.3）**

（5）发病和患病登记/报告数据利用发布情况

各级疾控中心所在地开展恶性肿瘤、脑卒中和心肌梗死病例报告的数据，以编写年报的形式发布及利用信息为主，其比例分别为61.1%、60.4%与60.4%，与2009年相比略有增加（图2-44）。

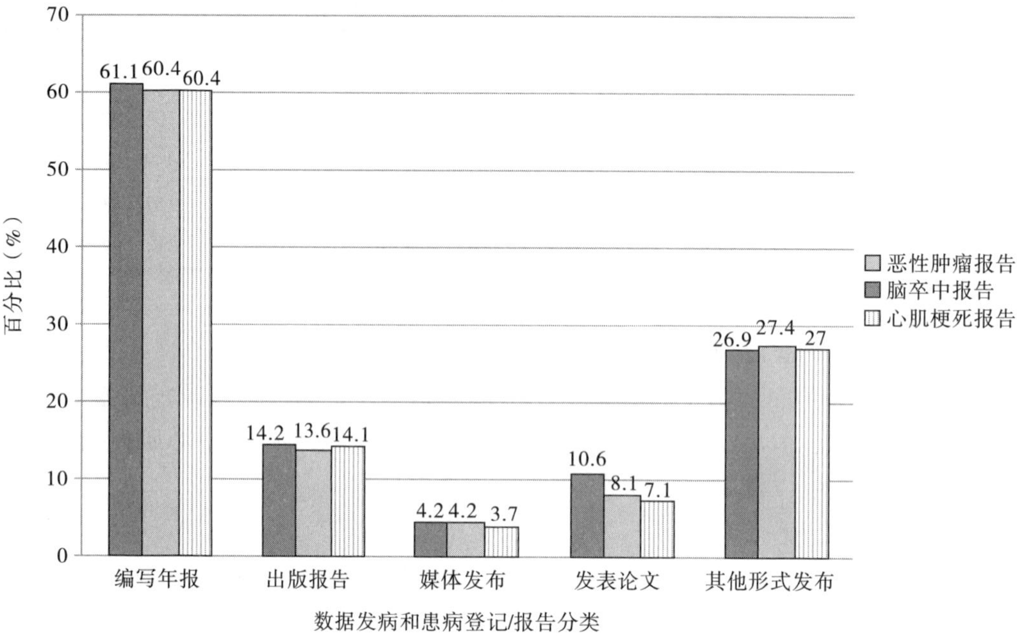

图 2-44 各类慢性病发病和患病报告/登记数据信息发布及利用情况

（6）发病和患病登记/报告的信息被采纳的情况

各地、各级疾控中心开展恶性肿瘤、脑卒中与心肌梗死病例报告的信息被采纳的比例分别为63.8%、65.6%、65.7%，省级疾控中心开展恶性肿瘤病例报告信息被采纳的比例高于地市级与县（区）级疾控中心，而脑卒中与心肌梗死病例报告的信息被采纳的比例均以县（区）级疾控中心为最高。从地区分布来看，东部地区开展恶性肿瘤、脑卒中与心肌梗死病例报告的信息被采纳的比例高于中、西部地区（表2-75、表2-76）。

表 2-75 各级疾控中心所在地开展恶性肿瘤、脑卒中和心肌梗死病例报告的信息被采纳的比例［机构数（%）］

级别	恶性肿瘤	脑卒中	心肌梗死
省级	20（69.0）	7（53.8）	6（50.0）
地市级	109（64.9）	51（58.6）	49（59.0）
县（区）级	622（63.4）	426（66.8）	405（66.9）
合计	**751（63.8）**	**484（65.6）**	**460（65.7）**

表 2-76 不同地区疾控中心所在地开展恶性肿瘤、脑卒中和心肌梗死病例报告的信息被采纳的比例［机构数（%）］

地区	恶性肿瘤	脑卒中	心肌梗死
东部	372（65.3）	257（71.8）	246（71.9）
中部	178（61.0）	101（57.7）	97（57.1）
西部	201（63.6）	126（61.5）	117（62.2）
合计	**751（63.8）**	**484（65.6）**	**460（65.7）**

2. 基层医疗卫生机构开展发病和患病登记报告的情况

各地被调查基层医疗卫生机构开展新发脑卒中病例报告工作的比例为 27.1%（2009 年，18.6%），其中社区卫生服务中心的比例为 36.9%，乡镇卫生院为 17.4%，均高于 2009 年（27.4%、9.5%）；开展急性心肌梗死病例报告的比例为 23.8%（2009 年，13.0%），其中社区卫生服务中心的比例为 32.5%，乡镇卫生院为 15.1%，均高于 2009 年（18.7%、7.0%）。

东、中、西部地区开展新发脑卒中病例报告的比例分别为 39.2%、18.3%与 20.5%，均高于 2009 年（31.1%、14.9%、6.5%）；开展急性心肌梗死病例报告的比例分别为 35.5%、15.9%与 16.8%，均高于 2009 年（21.7%、9.4%、5.4%）（表 2-77、表 2-78）。

表 2-77 各地基层医疗卫生机构开展新发脑卒中病例报告情况［机构数（%）］

机构分类	东部	中部	西部	合计
乡镇卫生院	98（26.3）	65（13.9）	94（14.7）	257（17.4）
社区卫生服务中心	350（45.4）	81（24.5）	114（30.3）	545（36.9）
合计	**448（39.2）**	**146（18.3）**	**208（20.5）**	**802（27.1）**

表 2-78 各地基层医疗卫生机构开展急性心肌梗死病例报告情况［机构数（%）］

机构分类	东部	中部	西部	合计
乡镇卫生院	88（23.7）	59（12.6）	76（11.9）	223（15.1）
社区卫生服务中心	318（41.3）	68（20.5）	94（25.0）	480（32.5）
合计	**406（35.5）**	**127（15.9）**	**170（16.8）**	**703（23.8）**

七、慢性病干预与管理能力

慢性病干预主要指采取各种措施，控制慢性病和相关危险因素流行，促进慢性病的早期发现和规范管理或延缓慢性病及并发症的发生和发展。慢性病干预与管理工作主要包括三个环节，即危险因素控制、早诊早治和规范化管理。

慢性病干预与管理能力主要指各级各地开展危险因素控制、慢性病患者和高危人群早发现、管理及康复等工作的情况。

（一）主要慢性病及其高危人群的危险因素干预情况

各级疾控中心开展或参与慢性病高危人群个体化干预的比例为 28.1%较 2009 年有所上升（13.7%），开展或参与 6 种主要慢性病患者个体化干预工作的各级疾控中心机构比例从高到低，分别为高血压 64.1%、糖尿病 62.8%、恶性肿瘤 21.4%、脑卒中 15.1%、冠心病 14.3%和慢性呼吸系统疾病 8.7%，较 2009 年均有提高，（2009 年分别为 36.1%、32.2%、16.1%、10.9%、11.0%、6.5%）。

省、地市、县（区）开展恶性肿瘤患者和高危人群个体化干预工作的机构比例呈下降趋势，省、地市和县（区）开展冠心病、慢性呼吸系统疾病患者个体化干预工作的机构比例则呈上升趋势。开展高血压、脑卒中患者个体化干预工作的省级比例高于县（区）级，地市级开展比例最低，开展糖尿病患者个体化干预工作的比例以县区级最高，省级次之，地市级最低（表 2-79）。慢性呼吸系统疾病干预工作开展比例呈东、中、西部上升趋势，高危人群干预工作呈东、中、西部下降趋势，其他慢性病患者干预工作开展比例均为东部最高，西部其次，中部最低（表 2-80）。

表 2-79 各级疾控中心开展或参与慢性病患者及高危人群干预工作的情况 [机构数（%）]

级别	高血压	糖尿病	恶性肿瘤	脑卒中	冠心病	慢性呼吸系统疾病	高危人群
省级	23（71.9）	20（62.5）	10（31.3）	5（15.6）	3（9.4）	2（6.3）	15（46.9）
地市级	199（57.5）	191（55.2）	74（21.4）	43（12.4）	40（11.6）	29（8.4）	112（32.4）
县（区）级	1904（64.8）	1872（63.7）	627（21.3）	452（15.4）	431（14.7）	258（8.8）	803（27.3）
合计	2126（64.1）	2083（62.8）	711（21.4）	500（15.1）	474（14.3）	289（8.7）	930（28.1）

表 2-80　各地区疾控中心开展或参与慢性病患者及高危人群干预工作的情况 [机构数（%）]

地区	高血压	糖尿病	恶性肿瘤	脑卒中	冠心病	慢性呼吸系统疾病	高危人群
东部	706（71.1）	691（69.6）	308（31.0）	226（22.8）	199（20.0）	67（6.7）	347（34.9）
中部	604（60.7）	595（59.8）	157（15.8）	106（10.7）	103（10.4）	85（8.5）	256（25.7）
西部	816（61.5）	797（60.1）	246（18.5）	168（12.7）	172（13.0）	137（10.3）	327（24.6）
合计	**2126（64.1）**	**2083（62.8）**	**711（21.4）**	**500（15.1）**	**474（14.3）**	**289（8.7）**	**930（28.1）**

慢性病相关危险因素主要包括 4 种行为危险因素，如烟草使用、不合理膳食、身体活动不足与有害饮酒；4 种生物危险因素，如超重肥胖、高血压、血糖升高、血脂异常。2011 年全国分别有 35.2%、24.7%、20.7%、16.2%的疾控中心开展了烟草使用、膳食、身体活动、酒精使用的相关干预项目或工作，较 2009 年疾控中心开展这四项目干预工作的比例明显升高（2009 年分别为 18.4%、15.4%、12.2%和 9.3%）。相较 2009 年，三级开展烟草相关项目或工作的比例均有所提高。开展膳食、身体活动和酒精使用相关项目的地市和县区级比例均提高，省级比例下降。2011 年，省级疾控中心开展烟草使用、膳食、身体活动、酒精使用的相关干预项目或工作的比例高于地市级与县（区）级。从地区分布来看，开展烟草使用、身体活动、酒精使用相关干预项目或工作的比例呈东、中、西下降趋势。

2011 年全国分别有 20.2%、33.4%、31.8%、16.2%的疾控中心开展了超重肥胖、高血压、高血糖、血脂异常相关的干预项目或工作，较 2009 年疾控中心开展这四项干预工作的比例明显升高（2009 年分别是 11.5%、19.9%、17.2%、9.9%）。相较 2009 年，地市级和县（区）级开展这四项工作的比例均有所上升，省级比例反而下降。2011 年，省级疾控中心开展超重肥胖、高血压、血糖升高、血脂异常相关的干预项目或工作的比例高于地市级与县（区）级。从地区分布来看，东部地区开展的比例高于中、西部地区。

2007 年 9 月 1 日，原卫生部启动全民健康生活方式行动。从本次调查结果来看，全国 52.2%的疾控中心开展了全民健康生活方式行动，其中有 30 个省级开展了全民健康生活方式行动，开展比例为 93.8%；地市级的开展比例为 68.2%；县区级的开展比例为 49.9%。从地区分布来看，东部地区最高为 64.0%，其次是中部（55.1%），西部地区比例最低为 41.2%（表 2-81 和表 2-82）。

表 2-81 各级疾控中心开展或参与慢性病相关危险因素控制工作的情况 [机构数（%）]

级别	全民健康生活方式	烟草	膳食	身体活动	酒精使用	超重肥胖	血压	血糖	血脂
省级	30（93.8）	27（84.4）	12（37.5）	10（31.3）	7（21.9）	9（28.1）	11（34.4）	11（34.4）	4（12.5）
地市级	236（68.2）	160（46.2）	84（24.3）	78（22.5）	55（15.9）	65（18.8）	94（27.2）	93（26.9）	58（16.8）
县（区）级	1465（49.9）	981（33.4）	724（24.7）	598（20.4）	475（16.2）	594（20.2）	1001（34.1）	950（32.3）	475（16.2）
合计	1731（52.2）	1168（35.2）	820（24.7）	686（20.7）	537（16.2）	668（20.2）	1106（33.4）	1054（31.8）	537（16.2）

表 2-82 各地疾控中心开展或参与慢性病相关危险因素控制工作的情况 [机构数（%）]

级别	全民健康生活方式	烟草	膳食	身体活动	酒精使用	超重肥胖	血压	血糖	血脂
东部	636（64.0）	412（41.5）	268（27.0）	243（24.5）	187（18.8）	239（24.1）	369（37.2）	349（35.1）	191（19.2）
中部	548（55.1）	364（36.6）	279（28.0）	204（20.5）	159（16.0）	195（19.6）	303（30.5）	292（29.3）	136（13.7）
西部	547（41.2）	392（29.5）	273（20.6）	239（18.0）	191（14.4）	234（17.6）	434（32.7）	413（31.1）	210（15.8）
合计	1731（52.2）	1168（35.2）	820（24.7）	686（20.7）	537（16.2）	668（20.2）	1106（33.4）	1054（31.8）	537（16.2）

（二）慢性病患者早发现及高危人群早发现工作情况

1. 开展 35 岁以上居民首诊测血压工作的情况

2011 年，94.1%的基层医疗卫生机构开展了 35 岁以上居民首诊测血压工作，其中 96.5%的社区卫生服务中心和 91.7%的乡镇卫生院开展了此项工作，均比 2009 年有所提高（2009 年分别是 89.1%与 43.8%）。社区卫生服务中心和乡镇卫生院首诊测血压的年平均服务人数分别为 10049.2 人与 6524.6 人，较 2009 年明显上升（2009 年，分别是 8424.5 人与 3742.9 人）。

2011 年基层医疗卫生机构开展 35 岁以上居民首诊测血压工作的比例，东、中、西部乡镇卫生院分别为 94.4%、92.1%、89.8%，较 2009 年（分别为 50.0%、43.0%、40.9%）明显上升。社区卫生服务中心开展首诊测血压的比例东、中、西部分别为 97.0%、96.1%、95.7%，较 2009 年（分别为 90.3%、87.3%、88.4%）有所上升。基层医疗卫生机构开展首诊测血压年均服务人数，东部最高、中部其次、西部最低（图 2-45、图 2-46）。

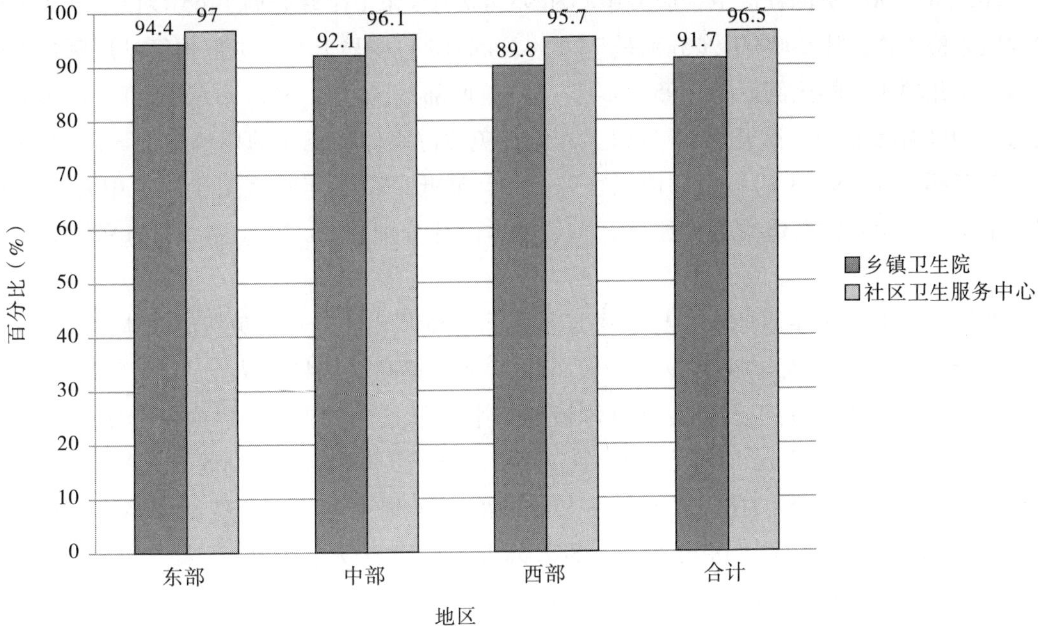

图 2-45 各地区基层医疗卫生机构开展 35 岁以上居民首诊测血压工作的机构情况（%）

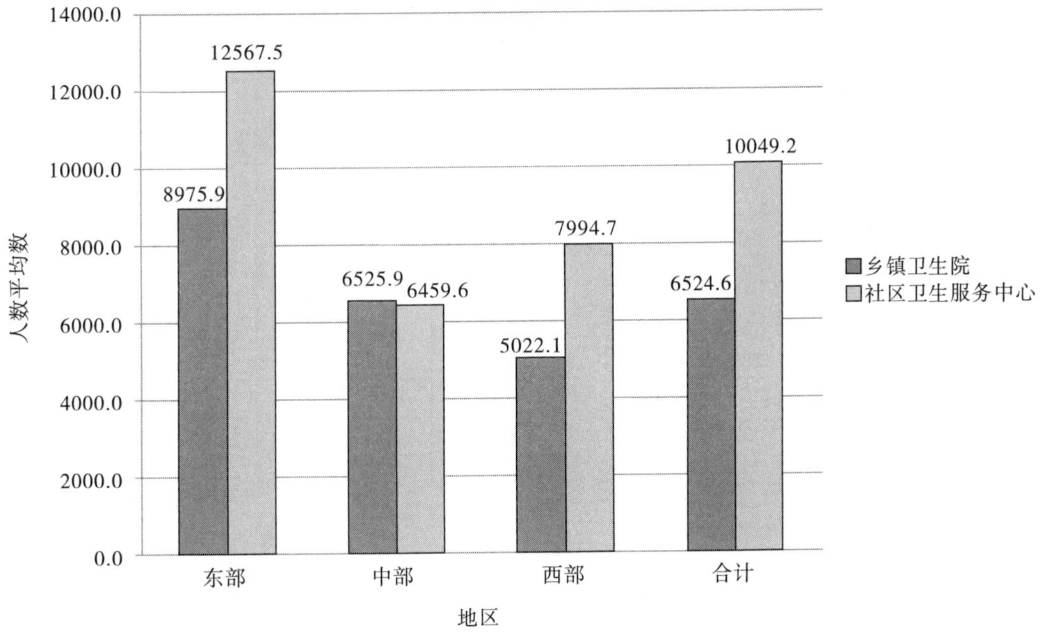

图 2-46 各地基层医疗卫生机构开展 35 岁以上居民首诊测血压工作的平均服务人数

2. 开展 65 岁以上老年人免费健康体检工作情况

2011 年，90. 9%的社区卫生服务中心和 93. 4%的乡镇卫生院开展了 65 岁以上老年人免费健康体检工作，比 2009 年（分别是 74. 8%、45. 0%）明显上升，中部地区基层医疗卫生机构开展此项工作的比例最高（95. 1%），其次是西部地区（91. 8%），东部地区（90. 4%）最低。2011 年乡镇卫生院开展 65 岁以上老年人免费健康体检工作的比例中部最高 95. 3%，其次是东部地区（93. 8%），西部地区（91. 7%）最低。2011 年社区卫生服务中心开展 65 岁以上老年人免费健康体检工作比例，东、中、西部分别是 88. 7%、94. 9%与 92. 0%（图 2-47）。

2011 年，社区卫生服务中心与乡镇卫生院开展 65 岁以上老年人免费健康体检的平均服务人数分别是 2420. 6 人与 2006. 9 人，较 2009 年有所提高（1744. 1 人与 1235. 5 人）。乡镇卫生院开展 65 岁以上老年人免费健康体检的年平均服务人数东、中、西部分别是 2637. 9 人、2225. 8 人、1459. 3 人，均较 2009 年（1547. 2 人、1307. 6 人、1008. 6 人）明显升高，分布趋势与 2009 年一致。社区卫生服务中心开展 65 岁以上老年人免费健康体检的年平均服务人数东、中、西部地区分别是 2887. 1 人、1717. 0 人、2136. 3 人，均较 2009 年（2235. 7 人、1282. 9 人、1047. 4 人）明显上升（图 2-48）。

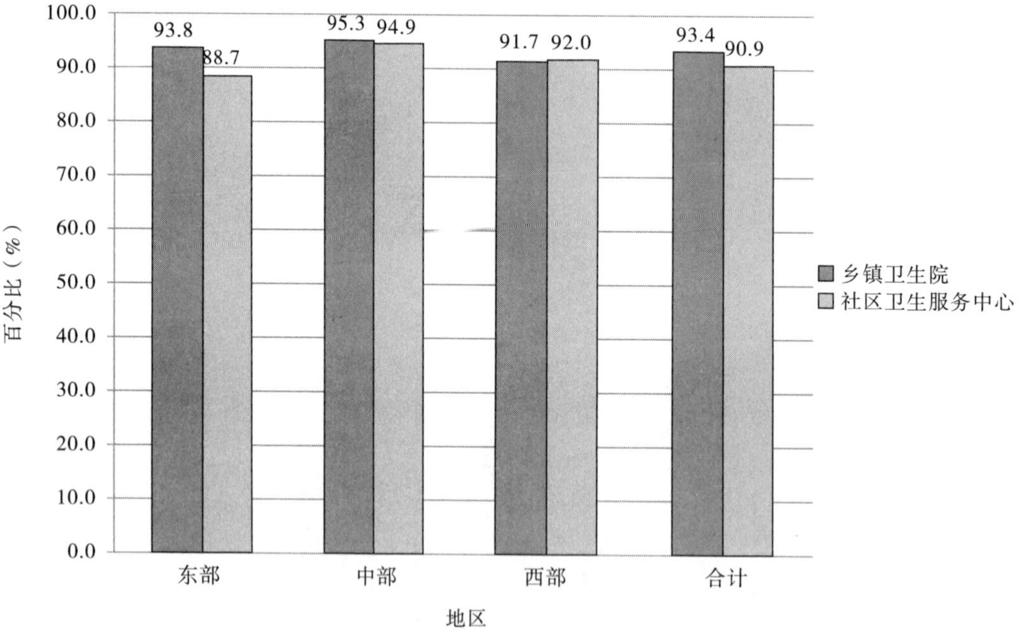

图 2-47 各地区基层医疗卫生机构开展 65 岁以上老年人免费健康体检工作的情况

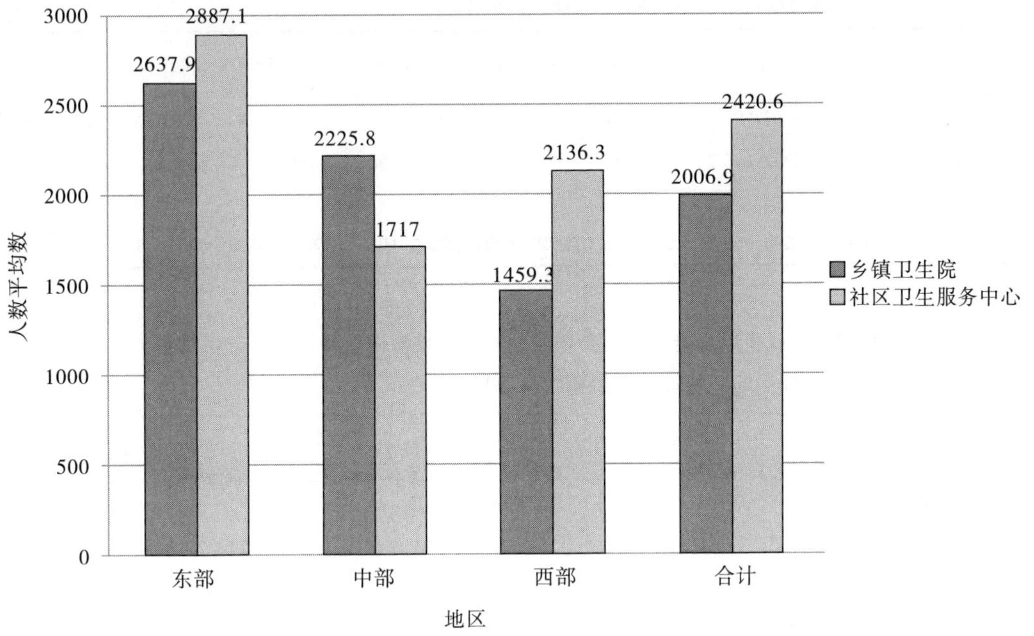

图 2-48　各地区基层医疗卫生机构开展 65 岁以上老年人免费健康体检工作的平均服务人数

2011 年在开展 65 岁以上老年人免费健康体检的基层医疗卫生机构中，各项检查项目开展的比例从高到低依次为，血压（99.9%）、体重（98.8%）、身高（98.7%）、血糖（95.5%）、腰围（93.0%）、心电图检查（80.9%）、血脂（64.9%）、X 线检查（36.6%）。开展血糖、腰围、心电图检查和血脂检查项目的比例分别较 2009 年有所上升。社区卫生服务中心开展各项检查项目的比例从高到低依次为血压（99.9%）、血糖（98.7%）、体重（98.3%）、身高（98.2%）、腰围（91.2%）、心电图检查（90.4%）、血脂（77.5%）、X 线检查（41.1%），社区卫生服务中心开展血糖、血脂、X 线与心电图检查的比例高于乡镇卫生院，而其他检查如血压、身高、体重、腰围的开展比例乡镇卫生院高于社区卫生服务中心，与 2009 年的情况不同，2009 年除体重测量一项外，社区卫生服务中心开展其他指标检查的比例均高于乡镇卫生院。从地区分布来看，2011 年基层医疗卫生机构开展的检查项目除血糖、血脂、X 线检查外，其余项目的开展比例均是西部地区高于中部地区、中部地区高于东部地区，血糖、血脂检测的开展比例是东部地区高于中部地区、中部地区高于西部地区，X 线检查的开展比例是东部地区最高，中、西部地区无差异（表 2-83、表 2-84）。

表 2-83 开展 65 岁以上老年人免费健康体检的两类被调查基层医疗卫生机构中各项检查项目的开展情况［机构数（%）］

机构	身高	体重	腰围	血压	血糖	血脂	X 线检查	心电图检查
乡镇卫生院	1368（99.2）	1369（99.3）	1306（94.7）	1378（99.9）	1274（92.4）	726（52.6）	443（32.1）	989（71.7）
社区卫生服务中心	1320（98.2）	1321（98.3）	1226（91.2）	1343（99.9）	1327（98.7）	1041（77.5）	553（41.1）	1215（90.4）
合计	2688（98.7）	2690（98.8）	2532（93.0）	2721（99.9）	2601（95.5）	2767（64.9）	996（36.6）	2204（80.9）

表 2-84 开展 65 岁以上老年人免费健康体检的各地被调查基层医疗卫生机构中各项检查项目的开展情况［机构数（%）］

地区	身高	体重	腰围	血压	血糖	血脂	X 线检查	心电图检查
东部	1008（97.6）	1009（97.7）	914（88.5）	1032（99.9）	1003（97.1）	773（74.8）	417（40.4）	892（86.4）
中部	753（99.2）	753（99.2）	720（94.9）	758（99.9）	734（96.7）	495（65.2）	259（34.1）	658（86.7）
西部	927（99.6）	928（99.7）	898（96.9）	931（100.0）	864（92.8）	499（53.6）	320（34.4）	654（70.2）
合计	2688（98.7）	2690（98.8）	2532（93.0）	2721（99.9）	2601（95.5）	2767（64.9）	996（36.6）	2204（80.9）

（三）主要慢性病患者及高危人群管理

1. 高血压患者与高危人群管理

2011 年，96.8%的被调查基层医疗卫生机构开展了高血压患者建档工作，明显高于 2009 年（62.8%）。44.0%的被调查基层医疗卫生机构开展了血压正常高值者建档工作，明显高于 2009 年（26.8%）。在东、中、西部，社区卫生服务中心开展高血压患者和血压正常高值者建档工作的比例均高于乡镇卫生院（表 2-85 和表 2-86）。

表 2-85 被调查基层医疗卫生机构开展高血压患者建档工作的情况［机构数（%）］

机构	东部	中部	西部	合计
乡镇卫生院	360（96.8）	449（96.2）	596（93.4）	1404（95.1）
社区卫生服务中心	762（98.8）	324（97.9）	369（98.1）	1455（98.4）
合计	1121（98.1）	773（96.9）	965（95.2）	2859（96.8）

表 2-86　被调查基层医疗卫生机构开展血压正常高值者建档工作的情况［机构数（%）］

机构	东部	中部	西部	合计
乡镇卫生院	132（35.5）	176（37.7）	253（39.7）	561（38.0）
社区卫生服务中心	384（49.8）	177（53.5）	177（47.1）	738（49.9）
合计	**516（45.1）**	**353（44.2）**	**430（43.4）**	**1299（44.0）**

在被调查基层医疗卫生服务机构中，分别有 96.0%和 34.3%开展了高血压患者随访管理和血压正常高值者随访管理工作。开展高血压患者随访管理工作的比例呈东、中、西部逐渐下降趋势，血压正常高值者随访管理工作开展比例东部地区最高，西部地区其次，中部地区最低（表 2-87 和表 2-88）。

表 2-87　被调查的基层医疗卫生机构中开展高血压患者随访管理工作的情况［机构数（%）］

机构	东部	中部	西部	合计
乡镇卫生院	360（96.8）	441（94.4）	588（92.2）	1389（94.0）
社区卫生服务中心	760（98.6）	321（97.0）	367（97.6）	1448（98.0）
合计	**1120（98.0）**	**762（95.5）**	**955（94.2）**	**2837（96.0）**

表 2-88　被调查的基层医疗卫生机构中开展血压正常高值者随访管理工作的情况［机构数（%）］

机构	东部	中部	西部	合计
乡镇卫生院	102（27.4）	127（27.2）	198（31.0）	427（28.9）
社区卫生服务中心	315（40.9）	124（37.5）	148（39.4）	587（39.7）
合计	**417（36.5）**	**251（31.5）**	**346（34.1）**	**1014（34.3）**

经调查并估算，开展高血压患者管理的基层医疗卫生机构所在辖区内，高血压患者的管理率为 14.2%，管理人群规范管理率为 82.6%，控制率为 53.1%（均比 2009 年调查数据有所提高，2009 年三者分别为 12.0%、73.8%和 48.7%）。社区卫生服务中心只有高血压患者的控制率高于乡镇卫生院。高血压患者管理率呈东、西、中部下降趋势；规范管理率西部地区最高，中部地区次之，东部最低；控制率东部最高、西部次之、中部最低（表 2-89 和表 2-90）。

表 2-89 被调查基层医疗卫生机构开展高血压患者管理工作的情况

机构	机构数	估计患者数（万人）	管理率（%）	规范管理率（%）	控制率（%）
乡镇卫生院	1389	1073.9	15.4	83.8	49.0
社区卫生服务中心	1448	1931.1	13.6	81.8	55.8
合计	2837	3005.0	14.2	82.6	53.1

表 2-90 各地区被调查基层医疗卫生机构开展高血压患者管理工作的情况

地区	机构数	估计患者数（万人）	管理率（%）	规范管理率（%）	控制率（%）
东部	1120	1208.5	19.7	81.9	53.8
中部	762	1076.6	9.9	83.3	51.5
西部	955	719.9	11.4	83.9	53.5
合计	2837	3005.0	14.2	82.6	53.1

2. 糖尿病患者与高危人群管理

2011 年，95.6%的被调查基层医疗卫生机构开展了糖尿病患者建档工作，28.2%的被调查基层医疗卫生机构开展了糖尿病高危人群即空腹血糖受损/糖耐量减低者建档工作，这两项工作的开展比例均较 2009 年有所提高，2009 年分别为 61.3%和 15.5%。在东、中、西地区，社区卫生服务中心开展糖尿病患者建档和空腹血糖受损/糖耐量减低者建档工作的比例均高于乡镇卫生院（表 2-91 和表 2-92）。

表 2-91 被调查基层医疗卫生机构开展糖尿病患者建档工作的情况［机构数（%）］

基层分类	东部	中部	西部	合计
乡镇卫生院	358（96.2）	442（94.7.）	573（89.8）	1373（93.0）
社区卫生服务中心	759（98.4）	325（98.2）	369（98.1）	1453（98.3）
合计	1117（97.7）	767（96.1）	942（92.9）	2826（95.6）

表 2-92 被调查基层医疗卫生机构开展糖尿病高危人群建档工作的情况 [机构数 (%)]

基层分类	东部	中部	西部	合计
乡镇卫生院	69 (18.6)	108 (23.1)	132 (20.7)	309 (20.9)
社区卫生服务中心	290 (37.6)	122 (36.9)	112 (29.8)	524 (35.5)
合计	**359 (12.1)**	**230 (28.8)**	**244 (24.1)**	**833 (28.2)**

在被调查基层医疗卫生服务机构中，分别有 94.7%和 23.9%开展了糖尿病患者随访管理与空腹血糖受损/糖耐量减低者随访管理工作。分地区比较，东部最高，中部其次，西部最低（表 2-93 和表 2-94）。

表 2-93 被调查基层医疗卫生机构开展糖尿病患者随访管理工作的情况 [机构数 (%)]

基层分类	东部	中部	西部	合计
乡镇卫生院	356 (95.7)	433 (92.7)	566 (88.7)	1355 (91.7)
社区卫生服务中心	755 (97.9)	322 (97.3)	367 (97.6)	1444 (97.7)
合计	**1111 (97.2)**	**755 (94.6)**	**933 (92.0)**	**2799 (94.7)**

表 2-94 被调查基层医疗卫生机构开展糖尿病高危人群随访管理工作的情况 [机构数 (%)]

基层分类	东部	中部	西部	合计
乡镇卫生院	61 (16.4)	93 (19.9)	111 (17.4)	265 (17.9)
社区卫生服务中心	243 (31.5)	98 (29.6)	99 (26.3)	440 (29.8)
合计	**304 (26.6)**	**191 (23.9)**	**210 (20.7)**	**705 (23.9)**

经调查并估算，开展糖尿病患者管理的基层医疗卫生机构所在辖区内，糖尿病患者管理率为 10.1%，管理人群规范管理率为 82.5%，控制率为 51.7%（2009 年，管理率、规范管理率和控制率分别为 7.9%、80.1%和 50.0%）。社区卫生服务中心所在辖区糖尿病患者的管理率、规范管理率及控制率均高于乡镇卫生院。糖尿病患者管理率和控制率东部地区最高、西部其次、中部最低；规范管理率呈东、中、西部下降趋势（表 2-95 和表 2-96）。

表 2-95 被调查基层医疗卫生机构开展糖尿病患者管理工作的情况（万人）

基层分类	机构数	估计患者数	管理率（%）	规范管理率（%）	控制率（%）
乡镇卫生院	1355（91.7）	427.48	9.0	82.1	47.0
社区卫生服务中心	1444（97.7）	784.06	10.7	82.7	53.8
合计	2799（94.7）	1211.55	10.1	82.5	51.7

表 2-96 各地区被调查基层医疗卫生机构开展糖尿病患者管理工作的情况（万人）

地区	机构数	估计患者数	管理率（%）	规范管理率（%）	控制率（%）
东部	1111	492.07	14.0	83.0	52.0
中部	755	431.79	6.9	82.1	50.6
西部	933	287.69	8.1	81.6	52.1
合计	2799	1211.55	10.1	82.5	51.7

（四）康复能力

慢性病康复服务能力主要指基层医疗卫生机构针对主要慢性病（如脑卒中）患者开展康复工作的情况。

2011 年，676 家被调查基层医疗卫生机构向脑卒中患者提供机械康复服务，占 22.9%，社区卫生服务中心和乡镇卫生院开展此项工作的比例分别为 38.6% 和 7.1%。2009 年 23.8%的被调查基层医疗卫生机构开展脑卒中患者康复工作，其中社区卫生服务中心与乡镇卫生院的比例分别为 43.0%与 3.9%。从地区分布来看，2011 年，东部地区开展脑卒中患者康复的比例最高（33.2%），其次是中部地区（20.6%）、最低为西部地区（13.1%），东中西部地区均是社区卫生服务中心开展脑卒中患者康复的比例高于乡镇卫生院（表 2-97）。

表 2-97 各地基层医疗卫生机构开展脑卒中患者康复工作的情况［机构数（%）］

基层分类	东部	中部	西部	合计
乡镇卫生院	53（14.3）	24（5.1）	28（4.4）	105（7.1）
社区卫生服务中心	326（42.3）	140（42.3）	105（28.0）	571（38.6）
合计	379（33.2）	164（20.6）	133（13.1）	676（22.9）

八、慢性病评估能力

慢性病评估能力主要指对慢性病流行情况及慢性病防控相关工作开展情况进行评估的能力。

2011年全国有30.6%的卫生行政部门或疾控中心对本辖区慢性病应对情况开展定期评估，比2009年的比例（13.3%）明显增高，省级的比例为37.5%，比2009年（40.6%）略有下降，地市与县（区）开展定期评估的比例比2009年（19.7%和12.2%）明显增加，从地区分布来看，东部地区比例最高，其次是西部地区、中部地区最低，2009年东部地区（21.7%）最高、中部地区（11.5%）次之、西部地区（8.3%）最低（表2-98）。

表2-98　各地、各级疾控中心或卫生行政部门对本辖区慢性病应对情况开展定期评估的情况［机构数（%）］

级别	东部	中部	西部	合计
省级	6（54.6）	2（25.0）	4（30.8）	12（37.5）
地市级	42（42.9）	23（22.1）	38（26.4）	103（29.8）
县（区）级	339（38.4）	227（25.7）	333（28.5）	899（30.6）
合计	**387（39.0）**	**252（25.3）**	**375（28.3）**	**1014（30.6）**

2011年全国各级疾控中心参与本辖区基层医疗卫生机构考核或评估的比例为71.1%，明显高于2009年的比例（40.9%），省级、地市级与县（区）级疾控中心参与本辖区基层医疗卫生机构考核或评估的比例分别为71.9%、70.8%和71.2%，均高于2009年各级疾控中心参与的比例（62.5%、45.1%、40.2%），东、中、西部地区疾控中心参与本辖区基层医疗卫生机构考核或评估的比例分别为81.0%、68.5%和65.7%，均较2009年（56.7%、40.6%、29.0%）显著增加（表2-99）。

表2-99　各地、各级疾控中心参与本辖区基层医疗卫生机构考核或评估的情况［机构数（%）］

级别	东部	中部	西部	合计
省级	9（81.8）	5（62.5）	9（69.2）	23（71.9）
地市级	76（77.6）	72（69.2）	97（67.4）	245（70.8）
县（区）级	719（81.3）	605（68.5）	766（65.5）	2090（71.2）
合计	**804（81.0）**	**682（68.5）**	**872（65.7）**	**2358（71.1）**

九、慢性病科研能力

慢性病科研能力主要指在慢性病防控领域开展科研工作的情况。

2011 年，全国 6.7%的疾控中心主持或参与了慢性病领域国内课题，略高于 2009 年（6.1%）的调查结果。省、地市、县（区）级疾控中心主持或参与慢性病领域国内课题的比例分别为 65.6%、15.0%、5.0%。在地区分布上，呈现东中西下降趋势，与 2009 年调查趋势（12.3%、3.6%、3.2%）一致（表 2-100）。

表 2-100　各地、各级疾控中心主持或参与慢性病领域国内科研课题的情况［机构数（%）］

级别	东部	中部	西部	合计
省级	9（81.8）	6（75.0.）	6（46.2）	21（65.6）
地市级	29（29.6）	10（9.7）	13（9.0）	52（15.0）
县（区）级	91（10.3）	32（3.6）	25（2.2）	148（5.0）
合计	**129（13.0）**	**48（4.8）**	**44（3.3）**	**221（6.7）**

2011 年，全国仅有 1.1%的疾控中心参与国际科研课题，低于 2009 年的调查结果（3.8%）。省、地市，县（区）级比例分别为 31.3%，2.0%和 0.7%，均低于 2009 年（46.9%、6.4%和 3.0%）。东、中、部地区分别为 2.2%、1.0%、0.4%，较 2009 年（4.1%、3.0%和 4.1%）有所下降（表 2-101）。

表 2-101　各地、各级疾控中心参与慢性病领域国际科研课题的情况［机构数（%）］

级别	东部	中部	西部	合计
省级	6（54.6.）	3（37.5）	1（7.7）	10（31.3）
地市级	4（4.1）	2（1.9）	1（0.7）	7（2.0）
县（区）级	12（1.4）	5（0.6）	3（0.3）	20（0.7）
合计	**22（2.2）**	**10（1.0）**	**5（0.4）**	**37（1.1）**

2011 年，全国仅有 8.3%的疾控中心有工作人员在国内外期刊发表过论文，略低于 2009 年的比例（9.7%）。省级 78.1%（与 2009 年持平），地市级 26.3%（略高于 2009 年的 25.1%），县（区）级 5.4%（低于 2009 年的 7.1%）。从地区看，东部地区 16.7%，中部 6.3%，西部 3.5%（表 2-102）。

表 2-102 各地、各级疾控中心工作人员在国内外期刊上发表论文的情况［机构数（%）］

级别	东部	中部	西部	合计
省级	11（100.0）	5（62.5）	9（69.2）	25（78.1）
地市级	39（39.8）	31（29.8）	21（14.6）	91（26.3）
县（区）级	116（13.1）	27（3.1）	16（1.4）	159（5.4）
合计	**166（16.7）**	**63（6.3）**	**46（3.5）**	**275（8.3）**

2011 年，全国仅有 27 个疾控中心出版过慢性病方面的专著，所占比例是 0.8%，低于 2009 年的比例（4.8%）。省级、地市级、县（区）级疾控中心出版慢性病方面专著的比例分别为 18.8%、2.0%和 0.5%，低于 2009 年的调查结果（21.9%、5.8%和 4.5%）。从地区分布看，东、中、西部分别为 1.4%、1.0%和 0.2%（表 2-103）。

表 2-103 各地各级疾控中心工作人员出版慢性病方面专著的情况［机构数（%）］

级别	东部	中部	西部	合计
省级	2（18.2）	2（25.0）	2（15.4）	6（18.8）
地市级	5（5.1）	2（1.9）	0（0.0）	7（2.0）
县（区）级	7（0.8）	6（0.7）	1（0.1）	14（0.5）
合计	**14（1.4）**	**10（1.0）**	**3（0.2）**	**27（0.8）**

2011 年，全国获科技进步奖的疾控中心有 27 个，占 0.8%。省、地市、县（区）三级机构所占比例依次降低，分别为 12.5%、3.8%和 0.3%［2009 年，省、地市和县（区）级的比例分别为 12.5%、5.8%和 2.7%］。从地区分布看，东、中、西部也依次降低，分别为 1.8%、0.5%、0.3%（表 2-104）。

表 2-104 各地各级疾控中心在慢性病研究领域获得科技进步奖的情况［机构数（%）］

级别	东部	中部	西部	合计
省级	3（27.3）	1（12.5）	0（0.0）	4（12.5）
地市级	8（8.2）	2（1.9）	3（2.1）	13（3.8）
县（区）级	7（0.8）	2（0.2）	1（0.1）	10（0.3）
合计	**18（1.8）**	**5（0.5）**	**4（0.3）**	**27（0.8）**

十、慢性病防控综合能力

本次报告在分模块分析各级各地慢性病防控能力的基础上，首次尝试对慢性病防控综合能力进行分析评估。

（一）综合评估概况

从之前评估的 8 个模块中选取 20 个核心指标（表 2-105），建立慢性病防控能力综合评估指标体系，每个指标赋值 5 分，共 100 分。根据各省（自治区、直辖市）各指标完成情况，对其慢性病防控综合能力进行评分并排序。

表 2-105　20 个核心指标在各个模块中的分布及赋值情况

模块	指标	单个指标赋值	模块内指标合计赋值
政策能力	政府慢性病防控专项财政经费配置情况	5	15
	是否有慢性病防控为主题的提案或议案	5	
	制定慢性病防控综合规划（政府或多部门制定）的情况	5	
基础配置能力	专门慢性病防控科设置情况	5	15
	专职慢性病防控人员占疾控卫生技术人员的比例	5	
	基层医疗卫生机构同时配置血糖仪和血压计的情况	5	
教育培训和指导能力	主办慢性病防控相关培训班的情况	5	15
	县（区）级疾控对基层医疗卫生机构开展指导的情况	5	
	基层医疗卫生机构举办健康讲座的情况	5	
合作能力	疾控机构与媒体合作的情况	5	10
	开展多部门合作的情况	5	
早期发现与监测能力	开展全人群死因监测的情况	5	15
	开展危险因素监测的情况	5	
	基层医疗卫生机构开展 35 岁以上首诊测血压的情况	5	

续　表

模块	指标	单个指标赋值	模块内指标合计赋值
干预与管理能力	开展全民健康生活方式行动的情况	5	20
	基层医疗卫生机构管理的高血压患者血压控制情况	5	
	基层医疗卫生机构管理的糖尿病患者血糖控制情况	5	
	基层医疗卫生机构同时开展高血压和糖尿病患者双向转诊的情况	5	
评估能力	疾控参与基层医疗卫生机构考核或评估的情况	5	5
科研能力	疾控慢性病防控人员发表论文的情况	5	5
合计		100	100

指标 1：政府慢性病防控专项财政经费配置情况

1. 来源

政策能力模块。

2. 分值

5 分。其中省、地市、县（区）三级所占比重分别为 4∶2∶4；直辖市中市和县（区）两级所占比重分别为 4∶6。

3. 指标含义

2011 年省、地市和县（区）各省（自治区、直辖市）三级政府是否配置慢性病防控专项经费。

4. 赋值方法

省级赋值，省级配置慢性病防控专项经费则赋值 2 分，没有配置则为 0 分；地市级赋值 = 1×本省内配置慢性病防控专项经费的地市级政府的比例；县（区）级赋值 = 2×本省内配置慢性病防控专项经费的县（区）级政府的比例。直辖市因没有地市一级，其赋值情况略有不同，直辖市级赋值与省（自治区）级一致；县（区）级赋值 = 3×本直辖市内配置慢性病防控专项经费的县（区）级政府的比例。

5. 各省（自治区、直辖市）得分及排序情况

各省（自治区、直辖市）综合评估指标 1 得分及排序情况见表 2-106。

表 2-106 各省（自治区、直辖市）“政府配置慢性病防控专项财政经费”指标得分及排序情况

省（市、区）	省级		地市级		县（区）级		合计得分	排序
	机构	得分	比例（%）	得分	比例（%）	得分		
北京	1	2	—	—	55.6	1.67	3.67	2
天津	1	2	—	—	27.8	0.83	2.83	6
河北	1	2	36.4	0.36	13.1	0.26	2.63	9
山西	0	0	18.2	0.18	17.7	0.35	0.53	24
内蒙古	0	0	8.3	0.08	7.1	0.14	0.22	30
辽宁	1	2	42.9	0.43	21.9	0.44	2.87	5
吉林	1	2	11.1	0.11	16.1	0.32	2.43	12
黑龙江	1	2	15.4	0.15	11.4	0.23	2.38	14
上海	1	2	—	—	83.3	2.50	4.50	1
江苏	1	2	61.5	0.62	45.1	0.90	3.52	3
浙江	0	0	63.6	0.64	36.4	0.73	1.36	20
安徽	1	2	25.0	0.25	15.3	0.31	2.56	11
福建	1	2	33.3	0.33	12.8	0.26	2.59	10
江西	0	0	0.0	0.00	10.1	0.20	0.20	31
山东	1	2	23.5	0.24	20.6	0.41	2.65	8
河南	1	2	17.7	0.18	11.7	0.23	2.41	13
湖北	0	0	15.4	0.15	18.4	0.37	0.52	25
湖南	0	0	21.4	0.21	19.4	0.39	0.60	23
广东	0	0	52.4	0.52	35.9	0.72	1.24	21
广西	1	2	14.3	0.14	4 7	0.09	2.24	16
海南	1	2	0.0	0.00	40.0	0.80	2.80	7
重庆	1	2	—	—	39.5	1.18	3.18	4
四川	0	0	9.5	0.10	13.7	0.27	0.37	28
贵州	1	2	11.1	0.11	10.1	0.20	2.31	15
云南	0	0	12.5	0.13	11.6	0.23	0.36	29
西藏	1	2	0.0	0.00	6.1	0.12	2.12	18
陕西	0	0	10.0	0.10	19.4	0.39	0.49	27
甘肃	0	0	0.0	0.00	9.6	0.19	0.19	32
青海	1	2	0.0	0.00	5.0	0.10	2.10	19
宁夏	0	0	40.0	0.40	5.3	0.11	0.51	26
新疆	1	2	7.1	0.07	7.5	0.15	2.22	17
兵团	0	0	35.7	0.36	16.9	0.34	0.70	22

指标 2：是否有慢性病防控为主题的提案或议案

1. 来源

政策能力模块。

2. 分值

5 分。其中省、地市、县（区）三级所占比重分别为 4∶2∶4；直辖市中市级和县（区）级所占比重分别为 4∶6。

3. 指标含义

2011 年省、地市和县（区）三级政府两会上是否有以慢性病防控为主题的提案或议案。

4. 赋值方法

省级赋值，省级两会上有以慢性病防控为主题的提案或议案则赋值 2 分，没有则为 0 分；地市级赋值=1×本省内地市级两会上有慢性病防控提案或议案的比例；县（区）级赋值=2×本省内县区级两会上有慢性病防控提案或议案的比例。直辖市因没有地市一级，其赋值情况略有不同，直辖市级赋值与省（自治区）级一致；县区级赋值=3×本直辖市内各县区两会上有慢性病防控提案或议案的比例。

5. 各省（自治区、直辖市）得分及排序情况

各省（自治区、直辖市）综合评估指标 2 得分及排序情况见表 2-107。

表 2-107　各省（自治区、直辖市）“慢性病防控为主题的提案或议案”指标得分及排序情况

省（市、区）	省级		地市级		县（区）级		合计得分	排序
	机构	得分	比例（%）	得分	比例（%）	得分		
北京	1	2	—	—	27.8	0.83	2.83	3
天津	1	2	—	—	5.6	0.17	2.17	11
河北	1	2	18.2	0.18	2.8	0.06	2.24	10
山西	0	0	27.3	0.27	7.6	0.15	0.42	17
内蒙古	0	0	8.3	0.08	3.0	0.06	0.14	29
辽宁	1	2	42.9	0.43	5.7	0.11	2.54	5
吉林	0	0	22.2	0.22	3.6	0.07	0.29	18
黑龙江	0	0	15.4	0.15	1.5	0.03	0.18	22
上海	1	2	—	—	38.9	1.17	3.17	1
江苏	1	2	46.2	0.46	10.8	0.22	2.68	4
浙江	1	2	54.6	0.55	19.3	0.39	2.93	2
安徽	0	0	6.3	0.06	4.1	0.08	0.14	28
福建	1	2	33.3	0.33	4.7	0.09	2.43	7

续 表

省（市、区）	省级		地市级		县（区）级		合计得分	排序
	机构	得分	比例（%）	得分	比例（%）	得分		
江西	1	2	18.2	0.18	4.0	0.08	2.26	9
山东	0	0	41.2	0.41	9.9	0.20	0.61	16
河南	1	2	29.4	0.29	8.6	0.17	2.47	6
湖北	0	0	7.7	0.08	4.6	0.09	0.17	23
湖南	0	0	7.1	0.07	3.9	0.08	0.15	27
广东	1	2	19.1	0.19	10.7	0.21	2.40	8
广西	0	0	14.3	0.14	2.3	0.05	0.19	21
海南	0	0	0	0.00	0	0.00	0.00	31
重庆	0	0	—	—	21.1	0.63	0.63	15
四川	0	0	4.8	0.05	5.5	0.11	0.16	25
贵州	0	0	11.1	0.11	2.3	0.05	0.16	26
云南	0	0	18.8	0.19	2.3	0.05	0.23	19
西藏	0	0	0	0.00	3.0	0.06	0.06	30
陕西	0	0	10.0	0.10	6.5	0.13	0.23	20
甘肃	1	2	6.7	0.07	1.2	0.02	2.09	13
青海	1	2	0	0.00	2.5	0.05	2.05	14
宁夏	1	2	0	0.00	5.3	0.11	2.11	12
新疆	0	0	0	0.00	0	0.00	0.00	32
兵团	0	0	7.1	0.07	4.4	0.09	0.16	24

指标 3：制定慢性病防控综合规划（政府或多部门制定）的情况

1. 来源

政策能力模块。

2. 分值

5 分。其中省、地市、县（区）三级所占比重分别为 4∶2∶4；直辖市中市级和县（区）级所占比重分别为 4∶6。

3. 指标含义

2011 年，省、地市和县（区）三级是否有政府或多部门制定的慢性病防控综合规划。

4. 赋值方法

省级赋值，省级政府或多部门制定慢性病防控综合规划则赋值 2 分，没有则为 0 分；地市级赋值=1×本省内有地市级政府或多部门制定慢性病防控综合规划的比例；县（区）级赋值=2×本省内有县（区）级政府或多部门制定慢性病防控综合规划的比例。直辖市因没有地市一级，其赋值情况略有不同，直辖市级赋值与省（自治区）级一致；县（区）级赋值=3×本直辖市内有县（区）级政府或多部门制定慢性病防控综合规划的比例。

5. 各省（自治区、直辖市）得分及排序情况

各省（自治区、直辖市）综合评估指标3得分及排序情况见表2-108。

表2-108 各省（自治区、直辖市）“政府或多部门制定慢性病防控综合规划”指标得分及排序情况

省（市、区）	省级		地市级		县（区）级		合计得分	排序
	机构	得分	比例（%）	得分	比例（%）	得分		
北京	0	0	—	—	22.2	0.67	0.67	5
天津	0	0	—	—	5.6	0.17	0.17	15
河北	0	0	0.0	0.00	4.0	0.08	0.08	24
山西	1	2	0.0	0.00	4.2	0.08	2.08	3
内蒙古	0	0	0.0	0.00	1.0	0.02	0.02	31
辽宁	0	0	0.0	0.00	4.8	0.10	0.10	22
吉林	0	0	0.0	0.00	10.7	0.21	0.21	10
黑龙江	0	0	0.0	0.00	2.3	0.05	0.05	28
上海	1	2	—	—	66.7	2.00	4.00	1
江苏	0	0	7.7	0.08	24.3	0.49	0.56	6
浙江	0	0	0.0	0.00	9.1	0.18	0.18	14
安徽	0	0	0.0	0.00	8.2	0.16	0.16	16
福建	0	0	0.0	0.00	3.5	0.07	0.07	25
江西	0	0	0.0	0.00	2.0	0.04	0.04	30
山东	0	0	0.0	0.00	6.4	0.13	0.13	19
河南	0	0	0.0	0.00	3.1	0.06	0.06	27
湖北	0	0	0.0	0.00	6.9	0.14	0.14	17
湖南	0	0	0.0	0.00	3.1	0.06	0.06	26
广东	0	0	0.0	0.00	9.7	0.19	0.19	13
广西	0	0	7.1	0.07	1.2	0.02	0.09	23
海南	0	0	0.0	0.00	10.0	0.20	0.20	12
重庆	0	0	—	—	36.8	1.11	1.11	4
四川	0	0	0.0	0.00	6.6	0.13	0.13	18
贵州	0	0	0.0	0.00	2.3	0.05	0.05	29
云南	1	2	0.0	0.00	5.4	0.11	2.11	2
西藏	0	0	0.0	0.00	0.0	0.00	0.00	32

续 表

省（市、区）	省级		地市级		县（区）级		合计得分	排序
	机构	得分	比例（%）	得分	比例（%）	得分		
陕西	0	0	0.0	0.00	10.2	0.20	0.20	11
甘肃	0	0	13.3	0.13	4.8	0.10	0.23	9
青海	0	0	0.0	0.00	5.0	0.10	0.10	21
宁夏	0	0	20.0	0.20	5.3	0.11	0.31	7
新疆	0	0	0	0.00	5.3	0.11	0.11	20
兵团	0	0	7.14	0.07	9.6	0.19	0.26	8

指标 4：专门慢性病防控科设置情况

1. 来源

基础配置能力模块。

2. 分值

5 分。其中省、地市、县（区）三级所占比重分别为 4∶2∶4；直辖市中市级和县（区）级所占比重分别为 4∶6。

3. 指标含义

2011 年，省、地市和县（区）三级疾控中心内是否设置专门承担慢性病防控工作的科（所）。

4. 赋值方法

省级赋值，省级疾控中心设置专门慢性病防控科（所）则赋值 2 分，没有则为 0 分；地市级赋值=1×本省内设置专门慢性病防控科（所）的地市级疾控中心的比例；县（区）级赋值=2×本省内设置专门慢性病防控科（所）的县区级疾控中心的比例。直辖市因没有地市一级，其赋值情况略有不同，直辖市级赋值与省（自治区）级一致；县（区）级赋值=3×本直辖市内设置专门慢性病防控科所的县（区）级疾控中心的比例。

5. 各省（自治区、直辖市）得分及排序情况

各省（自治区、直辖市）综合评估指标 4 得分及排序情况见表 2-109。

表 2-109　各省（自治区、直辖市）“疾控设置专门慢性病防控科所”指标得分及排序情况

省（市、区）	省级		地市级		县（区）级		合计得分	排序
	机构	得分	比例（%）	得分	比例（%）	得分		
北京	1	2	—	—	38.9	1.17	3.17	5
天津	1	2	—	—	44.4	1.33	3.33	3
河北	1	2	81.8	0.82	20.5	0.41	3.23	4

续　表

省（市、区）	省级		地市级		县（区）级		合计得分	排序
	机构	得分	比例（%）	得分	比例（%）	得分		
山西	1	2	63.6	0.64	19.3	0.39	3.02	7
内蒙古	1	2	66.7	0.67	15.2	0.30	2.97	9
辽宁	1	2	64.3	0.64	13.3	0.27	2.91	10
吉林	1	2	88.9	0.89	35.7	0.71	3.60	2
黑龙江	0	0	46.2	0.46	18.9	0.38	0.84	28
上海	1	2	—	—	77.8	2.33	4.33	1
江苏	1	2	46.2	0.46	21.6	0.43	2.89	11
浙江	1	2	45.5	0.45	14.8	0.30	2.75	12
安徽	1	2	25.0	0.25	4.1	0.08	2.33	19
福建	1	2	0.0	0.00	3.5	0.07	2.07	24
江西	1	2	18.2	0.18	2.0	0.04	2.22	22
山东	1	2	41.2	0.41	28.4	0.57	2.98	8
河南	0	0	58.8	0.59	23.9	0.48	1.07	26
湖北	1	2	61.5	0.62	20.7	0.41	3.03	6
湖南	1	2	14.3	0.14	7.0	0.14	2.28	21
广东	1	2	47.6	0.48	13.6	0.27	2.75	13
广西	1	2	14.3	0.14	0.0	0.00	2.14	23
海南	0	0	50.0	0.50	10.0	0.20	0.70	29
重庆	0	0	—	—	34.2	1.03	1.03	27
四川	1	2	19.1	0.19	8.7	0.17	2.37	18
贵州	0	0	11.1	0.11	6.7	0.13	0.25	30
云南	1	2	31.3	0.31	19.4	0.39	2.70	14
西藏	0	0	0.0	0.00	1.5	0.03	0.03	32
陕西	1	2	20.0	0.20	21.3	0.43	2.63	15
甘肃	1	2	13.3	0.13	9.6	0.19	2.33	20
青海	1	2	12.5	0.13	12.5	0.25	2.38	17
宁夏	1	2	0.0	0.00	0.0	0.00	2.00	25
新疆	1	2	42.9	0.43	5.3	0.11	2.54	16
兵团	0	0	7.1	0.07	2.9	0.06	0.13	31

指标5：专职慢性病防控人员占疾控中心卫生技术人员比例情况

1. 来源

基础配置能力模块。

2. 分值

5 分。其中省、地市、县（区）三级所占比重分别为 4∶2∶4；直辖市中市级和县（区）级所占比重分别为 4∶6。

3. 指标含义

2011 年，省、地市和县（区）三级疾控中心内专职慢性病防控在岗人员占疾控中心卫生技术在岗人员的比例。

4. 赋值方法

省、地市、县（区）专职慢性病防控在岗人员占疾控中心卫生技术在岗人员的理想比例分别为 5%、8%、10%。

（1）省级

卫生技术在岗人员数量=疾控中心在岗人员总数×78.4%（此比例由 2012 年卫生统计年鉴数据估算所得）。

专职人员占疾控中心卫生技术人员比例（以下简称“专职比例”）= 省级专职慢性病防控在岗人员数量/卫生技术在岗人员数量×100%。

专职比例≥5%，赋值 2 分；3.75%≤专职比例<5%，赋值 1.6 分；2.5%≤专职比例<3.75%，赋值 1.2 分；1.25%≤专职比例<2.5%，赋值 0.8 分；0<专职比例<1.25%，赋值 0.4 分；专职比例=0，赋值 0 分。

（2）地市级

卫生技术在岗人员数量=疾控中心在岗人员总数×81.3%（此比例由 2012 年卫生统计年鉴数据估算所得）。

专职人员占疾控中心卫生技术人员比例（以下简称“专职比例”）= 地市级专职慢性病防控在岗人员数量/卫生技术在岗人员数量×100%。

专职比例≥8%，赋值 1 分；6%≤专职比例<8%，赋值 0.8 分；4%≤专职比例<6%，赋值 0.6 分；2%≤专职比例<4%，赋值 0.4 分；0<专职比例<2%，赋值 0.2 分；专职比例=0，赋值 0 分。

（3）县（区）级

卫生技术在岗人员数量=疾控中心在岗人员总数×82.1%（此比例由 2012 年卫生统计年鉴数据计算所得）。

专职人员占疾控中心卫生技术人员比例（以下简称“专职比例”）= 县（区）级专职慢性病防控在岗人员数量/卫生技术在岗人员数量×100%。

专职比例≥10%，赋值 2 分；7.5%≤专职比例<10%，赋值 1.6 分；5%≤专职比例<7.5%，赋值 1.2 分；2.5%≤专职比例<5%，赋值 0.8 分；0<专职比例<2.5%，赋值 0.4 分；专职比例=0，赋值 0 分。

(4) 直辖市

直辖市市级赋值与省（自治区）级一致。县（区）级专职比例≥10%，赋值 3 分；7.5%≤专职比例<10%，赋值 2.4 分；5%≤专职比例<7.5%，赋值 1.8 分；2.5%≤专职比例<5%，赋值 1.2 分；0<专职比例<2.5%，赋值 0.6 分；专职比例=0，赋值 0 分。

5. 各省（自治区、直辖市）得分及排序情况

各省（自治区、直辖市）综合评估指标 5 得分及排序情况见表 2-110。

表 2-110 各省（自治区、直辖市）“专职慢性病防控人员占疾控中心卫生技术人员比例”指标得分及排序情况

省（市、区）	省级		地市级		县（区）级		合计得分	排序
	比例（%）	得分	比例（%）	得分	比例（%）	得分		
北京	2.2	0.8	—	—	3.9	1.2	2	18
天津	3.8	1.6	—	—	5.5	1.8	3.4	3
河北	5.6	2	3.3	0.4	3.8	0.8	3.2	4
山西	4.0	1.6	2.6	0.4	5.3	1.2	3.2	5
内蒙古	2.3	0.8	3.3	0.4	4.4	0.8	2	19
辽宁	4.6	1.6	3.0	0.4	2.7	0.8	2.8	8
吉林	3.2	1.2	4.3	0.6	3.5	0.8	2.6	12
黑龙江	4.2	1.6	3.4	0.4	4.2	0.8	2.8	9
上海	2.9	1.2	—	—	8.7	2.4	3.6	1
江苏	3.7	1.2	2.7	0.4	3.9	0.8	2.4	6
浙江	4.2	1.6	4.1	0.6	3.8	0.8	3	20
安徽	1.7	0.8	2.1	0.4	2.6	0.8	2	17
福建	3.9	1.6	1.8	0.2	1.2	0.4	2.2	21
江西	3.4	1.2	2.8	0.4	1.3	0.4	2	10
山东	3.9	1.6	3.0	0.4	3.8	0.8	2.8	22
河南	2.0	0.8	2.3	0.4	2.8	0.8	2	14
湖北	2.9	1.2	2.8	0.4	3.2	0.8	2.4	28
湖南	2.9	1.2	1.3	0.2	2.2	0.4	1.8	15
广东	2.7	1.2	3.0	0.4	4.1	0.8	2.4	23
广西	3.3	1.2	2.2	0.4	0.8	0.4	2	29
海南	1.2	0.4	2.9	0.4	4.0	0.8	1.6	30
重庆	1.0	0.4	—	—	4.4	1.2	1.6	25
四川	1.9	0.8	1.7	0.2	2.6	0.8	1.8	26
贵州	2.0	0.8	1.3	0.2	3.6	0.8	1.8	16

续 表

省（市、区）	省级		地市级		县（区）级		合计得分	排序
	比例（%）	得分	比例（%）	得分	比例（%）	得分		
云南	2.6	1.2	3.5	0.4	3.5	0.8	2.4	27
西藏	2.1	0.8	1.2	0.2	3.3	0.8	1.8	11
陕西	3.4	1.2	3.7	0.4	5.4	1.2	2.8	24
甘肃	2.1	0.8	3.4	0.4	4.8	0.8	2	2
青海	5.6	2	6.7	0.8	4.5	0.8	3.6	7
宁夏	3.8	1.6	4.1	0.6	2.9	0.8	3	31
新疆	2.0	0.8	2.0	0.4	1.5	0.4	1.6	32
兵团	0.0	0	1.4	0.2	5.0	1.2	1.4	18

指标 6：基层医疗卫生机构同时配置血糖仪和血压计的情况

1. 来源

基础配置能力模块。

2. 分值

5 分。

3. 指标含义

同时配置血糖仪和血压计的被调查基层医疗卫生机构比例。

4. 赋值方法

赋值=5×本省内同时配置血糖仪和血压计的被调查基层医疗卫生机构比例。

5. 各省（自治区、直辖市）得分及排序情况

各省（自治区、直辖市）综合评估指标 6 得分及排序情况见表 2-111。

表 2-111 各省（自治区、直辖市）“基层医疗卫生机构同时配置血糖仪和血压计”指标得分及排序情况

省（市、区）	基层配置血糖仪和血压计		排序
	比例（%）	得分	
北京	96.5	4.82	8
天津	100.0	5.00	1
河北	95.2	4.76	12
山西	90.5	4.52	24
内蒙古	84.2	4.21	28
辽宁	93.5	4.67	19

续 表

省（市、区）	基层配置血糖仪和血压计		排序
	比例（%）	得分	
吉林	94.4	4.72	13
黑龙江	96.3	4.82	9
上海	94.4	4.72	13
江苏	95.3	4.77	11
浙江	97.6	4.88	7
安徽	98.4	4.92	6
福建	98.9	4.95	4
江西	93.6	4.68	17
山东	93.4	4.67	20
河南	82.9	4.15	29
湖北	94.3	4.71	15
湖南	79.8	3.99	31
广东	91.2	4.56	23
广西	93.6	4.68	17
海南	93.8	4.69	16
重庆	95.4	4.77	10
四川	85.7	4.29	27
贵州	93.0	4.65	21
云南	98.8	4.94	5
西藏	14.3	0.71	32
陕西	91.7	4.58	22
甘肃	87.2	4.36	26
青海	87.5	4.38	25
宁夏	100.0	5.00	1
新疆	82.0	4.10	30
兵团	100.0	5.00	1

指标7：主办慢性病防控相关培训班情况

1. 来源

教育培训和指导能力模块。

2. 分值

5分。其中省、地市、县（区）三级所占比重分别为4∶2∶4；直辖市中市级和县

（区）级所占比重分别为 4∶6。

3. 指标含义

2011 年，省、地市和县（区）三级疾控中心是否主办过慢性病防控相关培训班的。

4. 赋值方法

省级赋值，省级疾控中心主办过慢性病防控相关培训班则赋值 2 分，没有则为 0 分；地市级赋值 = 1×本省内主办过慢性病防控相关培训班的地市级疾控中心比例；县（区）级赋值 = 2×本省内主办过慢性病防控相关培训班的县（区）级疾控中心比例。直辖市因没有地市一级，其赋值情况略有不同，直辖市级赋值与省（自治区）级一致；县（区）级赋值 = 3×本直辖市内主办过慢性病防控相关培训班的县（区）级疾控中心比例。

5. 各省（自治区、直辖市）得分及排序情况

各省（自治区、直辖市）综合评估指标 7 得分及排序情况见表 2-112。

表 2-112 各省（自治区、直辖市）"主办慢性病防控相关培训班"指标得分及排序情况

省（市、区）	省级		地市级		县（区）级		合计得分	排序
	机构	得分	比例（%）	得分	比例（%）	得分		
北京	1	2	—	—	100.0	3.00	5.00	1
天津	1	2	—	—	83.3	2.50	4.50	10
河北	1	2	90.9	0.91	79.0	1.58	4.49	11
山西	1	2	54.6	0.55	62.2	1.24	3.79	23
内蒙古	1	2	66.7	0.67	83.8	1.68	4.34	15
辽宁	1	2	100.0	1.00	72.4	1.45	4.45	13
吉林	1	2	100.0	1.00	87.5	1.75	4.75	6
黑龙江	1	2	69.2	0.69	59.1	1.18	3.87	21
上海	1	2	—	—	94.4	2.83	4.83	4
江苏	1	2	100.0	1.00	90.1	1.80	4.80	5
浙江	1	2	100.0	1.00	98.9	1.98	4.98	2
安徽	1	2	56.3	0.56	76.5	1.53	4.09	18
福建	1	2	77.8	0.78	30.2	0.60	3.38	29
江西	1	2	72.7	0.73	37.4	0.75	3.47	26
山东	1	2	82.4	0.82	81.6	1.63	4.45	12
河南	1	2	82.4	0.82	61.4	1.23	4.05	20
湖北	1	2	76.9	0.77	89.7	1.79	4.56	9
湖南	1	2	42.9	0.43	48.1	0.96	3.39	28
广东	1	2	90.5	0.90	76.7	1.53	4.44	14
广西	1	2	85.7	0.86	29.1	0.58	3.44	27

续 表

省（市、区）	省级		地市级		县（区）级		合计得分	排序
	机构	得分	比例（%）	得分	比例（%）	得分		
海南	1	2	100.0	1.00	95.0	1.90	4.90	3
重庆	1	2	—	—	89.5	2.68	4.68	8
四川	1	2	71.4	0.71	71.6	1.43	4.15	17
贵州	1	2	44.4	0.44	53.9	1.08	3.52	25
云南	1	2	56.3	0.56	74.4	1.49	4.05	19
西藏	1	2	0	0.00	16.7	0.33	2.33	32
陕西	1	2	60.0	0.60	87.0	1.74	4.34	16
甘肃	1	2	53.3	0.53	63.9	1.28	3.81	22
青海	1	2	37.5	0.38	70.0	1.40	3.78	24
宁夏	1	2	80.0	0.80	94.7	1.89	4.69	7
新疆	1	2	71.4	0.71	25.5	0.51	3.22	30
兵团	1	2	28.6	0.29	45.6	0.91	3.20	31

指标8：县（区）级疾控中心对基层医疗卫生机构开展指导的情况

1. 来源

教育培训和指导能力模块。

2. 分值

5分。

3. 指标含义

2011年对基层医疗卫生机构开展过慢性病防控相关指导的县（区）级疾控中心比例。

4. 赋值方法：赋值=5×本省（自治区、直辖市）内对基层医疗卫生机构开展过慢性病防控相关指导的县（区）级疾控中心比例。

5. 各省（自治区、直辖市）得分及排序情况

各省（自治区、直辖市）综合评估指标8得分及排序情况见表2-113。

表2-113 各省（自治区、直辖市）“县（区）级疾控中心对基层医疗卫生机构开展指导”指标得分及排序情况

省（市、区）	县（区）级疾控中心对基层开展指导		排序
	比例（%）	得分	
北京	61.1	3.06	8
天津	61.1	3.06	9

续 表

省（市、区）	县（区）级疾控中心对基层开展指导		排序
	比例（%）	得分	
河北	54.6	2.73	12
山西	45.4	2.27	20
内蒙古	38.4	1.92	25
辽宁	29.5	1.48	28
吉林	67.9	3.39	4
黑龙江	42.4	2.12	22
上海	94.4	4.72	1
江苏	67.6	3.38	5
浙江	78.4	3.92	2
安徽	54.1	2.70	14
福建	47.7	2.38	16
江西	27.3	1.36	29
山东	45.4	2.27	19
河南	46.6	2.33	17
湖北	64.4	3.22	6
湖南	46.5	2.33	18
广东	54.4	2.72	13
广西	41.9	2.09	23
海南	50.0	2.50	15
重庆	73.7	3.68	3
四川	58.5	2.92	11
贵州	37.1	1.85	26
云南	59.7	2.98	10
西藏	3.0	0.15	32
陕西	63.0	3.15	7
甘肃	38.6	1.93	24
青海	45.0	2.25	21
宁夏	31.6	1.58	27
新疆	20.2	1.01	30
兵团	11.8	0.59	31

指标 9：基层医疗卫生机构举办健康讲座的情况

1．来源

教育培训和指导能力模块。

2．分值

5 分。

3．含义

2011 年开展健康教育讲座的被调查基层医疗卫生机构的比例。

4．赋值方法：赋值 = 5×本省（自治区、直辖市）内开展健康教育讲座的被调查基层医疗卫生机构的比例。

5．各省（自治区、直辖市）得分及排序情况

各省（自治区、直辖市）综合评估指标 9 得分及排序情况见表 2-114。

表 2-114　各省（自治区、直辖市）“基层医疗卫生机构举办健康讲座”指标得分及排序情况

省（市、区）	基层医疗卫生机构举办健康讲座		排序
	比例（%）	得分	
北京	100.0	5.00	1
天津	94.2	4.71	12
河北	85.6	4.28	27
山西	89.3	4.46	20
内蒙古	82.1	4.11	29
辽宁	86.9	4.35	21
吉林	97.2	4.86	6
黑龙江	86.6	4.33	23
上海	98.6	4.93	5
江苏	99.5	4.98	2
浙江	95.8	4.79	9
安徽	96.0	4.80	8
福建	98.9	4.95	3
江西	79.5	3.97	30
山东	95.3	4.76	10
河南	90.2	4.51	18
湖北	96.2	4.81	7
湖南	86.8	4.34	22
广东	92.1	4.61	15
广西	90.3	4.52	17

续 表

省（市、区）	基层医疗卫生机构举办健康讲座		排序
	比例（%）	得分	
海南	93.8	4.69	13
重庆	98.9	4.94	4
四川	91.2	4.56	16
贵州	86.0	4.30	25
云南	95.1	4.75	11
西藏	7.1	0.36	32
陕西	89.8	4.49	19
甘肃	86.2	4.31	24
青海	68.8	3.44	31
宁夏	92.9	4.64	14
新疆	86.0	4.30	26
兵团	83.3	4.17	28

指标 10：疾控中心与媒体合作的情况

1. 来源

合作能力模块。

2. 分值

5 分。其中省、地市、县（区）三级所占比重分别为 4∶2∶4；直辖市中市级和县（区）级所占比重分别为 4∶6。

3. 指标含义

2011 年省、地市和县（区）三级疾控中心与媒体合作的比例。

4. 赋值方法

省级赋值，省级疾控中心与媒体开展合作则赋值 2 分，没有则为 0 分；地市级赋值 = 1 ×本省内与媒体合作的地市级疾控中心比例；县（区）级赋值 = 2×本省内与媒体合作的县（区）级疾控中心比例。直辖市因没有地市一级，其赋值情况略有不同，直辖市级赋值与省（自治区）级一致；县（区）级赋值 = 3×本直辖市内与媒体合作的县（区）级疾控中心比例。

5. 各省（自治区、直辖市）得分及排序情况

各省（自治区、直辖市）综合评估指标 10 得分及排序情况见表 2-115。

表 2-115 各省（自治区、直辖市）“与媒体合作”指标得分及排序情况

省（市、区）	省级		地市级		县（区）级		合计得分	排序
	机构	得分	比例（%）	得分	比例（%）	得分		
北京	1	2	—	—	88.9	2.67	4.67	1
天津	1	2	—	—	83.3	2.50	4.50	3
河北	1	2	81.8	0.82	36.9	0.74	3.56	8
山西	1	2	72.7	0.73	38.7	0.77	3.50	9
内蒙古	0	0	75.0	0.75	26.3	0.53	1.28	28
辽宁	0	0	100.0	1.00	24.8	0.50	1.50	25
吉林	0	0	66.7	0.67	30.4	0.61	1.27	29
黑龙江	1	2	53.9	0.54	39.4	0.79	3.33	13
上海	1	2	—	—	88.9	2.67	4.67	1
江苏	1	2	92.3	0.92	59.5	1.19	4.11	5
浙江	1	2	81.8	0.82	69.3	1.39	4.20	4
安徽	0	0	62.5	0.63	33.7	0.67	1.30	27
福建	0	0	66.7	0.67	22.1	0.44	1.11	30
江西	1	2	72.7	0.73	31.3	0.63	3.35	12
山东	1	2	94.1	0.94	50.4	1.01	3.95	6
河南	1	2	88.2	0.88	39.3	0.79	3.67	7
湖北	1	2	61.5	0.62	37.9	0.76	3.37	11
湖南	0	0	64.3	0.64	18.6	0.37	1.01	31
广东	1	2	52.4	0.52	43.7	0.87	3.40	10
广西	1	2	57.1	0.57	9.3	0.19	2.76	19
海南	0	0	100.0	1.00	25.0	0.50	1.50	25
重庆	0	0	—	—	68.4	2.05	2.05	24
四川	1	2	33.3	0.33	26.2	0.52	2.86	16
贵州	1	2	33.3	0.33	24.7	0.49	2.83	17
云南	0	0	31.3	0.31	15.5	0.31	0.62	32
西藏	1	2	0.0	0.00	3.0	0.06	2.06	23
陕西	1	2	30.0	0.30	34.3	0.69	2.99	14
甘肃	1	2	33.3	0.33	24.1	0.48	2.82	18
青海	1	2	12.5	0.13	10.0	0.20	2.33	22
宁夏	1	2	0.0	0.00	21.1	0.42	2.42	21
新疆	1	2	50.0	0.50	9.6	0.19	2.69	20
兵团	1	2	21.4	0.21	33.1	0.66	2.88	15

指标 11：开展多部门合作的情况

1. 来源

合作能力模块。

2. 分值

5 分。其中省、地市、县（区）三级所占比重分别为 4∶2∶4；直辖市中市级和县（区）级所占比重分别为 4∶6。

3. 指标含义

2011 年，省、地市和县（区）三级内至少有两家非卫生领域机构参与慢性病防控工作的地区比例。

4. 赋值方法

省级赋值，省级有两家以上非卫生领域机构参与慢性病防控工作则赋值 2 分，没有或不足两家则为 0 分；地市级赋值=1×有两家以上非卫生领域机构参与慢性病防控工作的地市级比例；县（区）级赋值=2×有两家以上非卫生领域机构参与慢性病防控工作的县（区）级疾控中心比例。直辖市因没有地市一级，其赋值情况略有不同，直辖市级赋值与省（自治区）级一致；县（区）级赋值=3×本直辖市内有两家以上非卫生领域机构参与慢性病防控工作的县（区）级疾控中心比例。

5. 各省（自治区、直辖市）得分及排序情况

各省（自治区、直辖市）综合评估指标 11 得分及排序情况见表 2-116。

表 2-116　各省（自治区、直辖市）“多部门合作”指标得分及排序情况

省（市、区）	省级		地市级		县（区）级		合计得分	排序
	机构	得分	比例（%）	得分	比例（%）	得分		
北京	0	0	—	—	27.8	0.83	0.83	10
天津	1	2	—	—	16.7	0.50	2.50	3
河北	0	0	9.1	0.09	4.6	0.09	0.18	23
山西	0	0	9.1	0.09	6.7	0.13	0.23	19
内蒙古	0	0	8.3	0.08	5.1	0.10	0.18	22
辽宁	0	0	14.3	0.14	2.9	0.06	0.20	20
吉林	1	2	33.3	0.33	10.7	0.21	2.55	2
黑龙江	0	0	0.0	0.00	6.8	0.14	0.14	27
上海	0	0	—	—	50.0	1.50	1.50	8
江苏	0	0	15.4	0.15	20.7	0.41	0.57	11
浙江	0	0	27.3	0.27	12.5	0.25	0.52	12
安徽	0	0	0.0	0.00	8.2	0.16	0.16	25

续 表

省（市、区）	省级		地市级		县（区）级		合计得分	排序
	机构	得分	比例（%）	得分	比例（%）	得分		
福建	0	0	22.2	0.22	4.7	0.09	0.32	14
江西	1	2	0.0	0.00	6.1	0.12	2.12	7
山东	1	2	29.4	0.29	15.6	0.31	2.61	1
河南	1	2	11.8	0.12	12.9	0.26	2.38	4
湖北	0	0	7.7	0.08	8.1	0.16	0.24	18
湖南	0	0	0.0	0.00	4.7	0.09	0.09	30
广东	0	0	9.5	0.10	8.7	0.17	0.27	16
广西	0	0	21.4	0.21	2.3	0.05	0.26	17
海南	0	0	0.0	0.00	5.0	0.10	0.10	29
重庆	0	0	—	—	39.5	1.18	1.18	9
四川	1	2	0.0	0.00	10.4	0.21	2.21	6
贵州	0	0	0.0	0.00	3.4	0.07	0.07	32
云南	0	0	6.3	0.06	5.4	0.11	0.17	24
西藏	0	0	0.0	0.00	4.6	0.09	0.09	31
陕西	0	0	0.0	0.00	9.3	0.19	0.19	21
甘肃	0	0	0.0	0.00	6.0	0.12	0.12	28
青海	0	0	0.0	0.00	7.5	0.15	0.15	26
宁夏	0	0	20.0	0.20	10.5	0.21	0.41	13
新疆	1	2	14.3	0.14	4.3	0.09	2.23	5
兵团	0	0	7.1	0.07	11.8	0.24	0.31	15

指标 12：开展全人群死因监测的情况

1. 来源

早期发现与监测能力模块。

2. 分值

5 分。

3. 指标含义

开展全死因监测的县（区）比例。

4. 赋值方法

据《中国慢性病防治工作规划（2012~2015 年）》要求到 2015 年全人群死因监测覆盖全国 90%的县（市、区）。

如省内开展全死因监测的县（区）比例≥90%，赋值 5 分；≥80%且<90%，赋值 4.5

分；≥70%且<80%，赋值 4 分；≥60%且<70%，赋值 3.5 分；≥50%且<60%，赋值 3 分；≥40%且<50%，赋值 2.5 分；≥30%且<40%，赋值 2 分；≥20%且<30%，则赋值 1.5 分；≥10%且<20%，则赋值 1 分；>0 且<10%，则赋值 0.5 分；=0，则赋值 0 分。

5. 各省（自治区、直辖市）得分及排序情况

各省（自治区、直辖市）综合评估指标 12 得分及排序情况见表 2-117。

表 2-117 各省（自治区、直辖市）“开展全人群死因监测”指标得分及排序情况

省（市、区）	开展全人群死因监测		排序
	比例（%）	得分	
北京	88.9	4.50	7
天津	94.4	5.00	4
河北	54.0	3.00	16
山西	52.9	3.00	17
内蒙古	51.5	3.00	19
辽宁	81.9	4.50	10
吉林	83.9	4.50	9
黑龙江	64.4	3.50	14
上海	94.4	5.00	5
江苏	94.6	5.00	3
浙江	96.6	5.00	2
安徽	42.9	2.50	25
福建	34.9	2.00	26
江西	26.3	1.50	28
山东	86.5	4.50	8
河南	50.3	3.00	22
湖北	48.3	2.50	23
湖南	54.3	3.00	15
广东	51.5	3.00	20
广西	14.0	1.00	30
海南	70.0	4.00	12
重庆	92.1	5.00	6
四川	51.4	3.00	21
贵州	7.9	0.50	31
云南	46.5	2.50	24
西藏	3.0	0.50	32

续　表

省（市、区）	开展全人群死因监测		排序
	比例（%）	得分	
陕西	25.0	1.50	29
甘肃	65.1	3.50	13
青海	80.0	4.50	11
宁夏	100.0	5.00	1
新疆	28.7	1.50	27
兵团	52.2	3.00	18

指标 13：开展危险因素监测的情况

1. 来源

早期发现与监测能力模块。

2. 分值

5 分。

3. 指标含义

2011 年除血脂以外其他各项危险因素监测都开展的县（区）比例。

4. 赋值方法

据《中国慢性病防治工作规划（2012~2015 年）》要求到 2015 年危险因素监测覆盖全国 50%的县（市、区）。

省内除血脂以外其他各项危险因素监测都开展的县区比例≥50%，则赋值 5 分；≥37.5%且<50%，则赋值 4 分；≥25%且<37.5%，则赋值 3 分；≥12.5%且<25%，则赋值 2 分；≥0 且<12.5%，则赋值 1 分；=0，则赋值 0 分。

5. 各省（自治区、直辖市）得分及排序情况

各省（自治区、直辖市）综合评估指标 13 得分及排序情况见表 2-118。

表 2-118　各省（自治区、直辖市）“开展危险因素监测”指标得分及排序情况

省（市、区）	开展全人群死因监测		排序
	比例（%）	得分	
北京	94.4	5.00	1
天津	66.7	5.00	3
河北	24.4	2.00	10
山西	10.9	1.00	23
内蒙古	21.2	2.00	11

续 表

省（市、区）	开展全人群死因监测		排序
	比例（%）	得分	
辽宁	20.0	2.00	12
吉林	33.9	3.00	7
黑龙江	15.9	2.00	14
上海	88.9	5.00	2
江苏	55.9	5.00	5
浙江	51.1	5.00	6
安徽	13.3	2.00	19
福建	9.3	1.00	26
江西	12.1	1.00	22
山东	26.2	3.00	9
河南	8.6	1.00	27
湖北	12.6	2.00	21
湖南	14.0	2.00	18
广东	28.2	3.00	8
广西	5.8	1.00	30
海南	15.0	2.00	16
重庆	57.9	5.00	4
四川	14.2	2.00	17
贵州	4.5	1.00	31
云南	6.2	1.00	29
西藏	3.0	1.00	32
陕西	13.0	2.00	20
甘肃	15.7	2.00	15
青海	7.5	1.00	28
宁夏	10.5	1.00	24
新疆	9.6	1.00	25
兵团	16.2	2.00	13

指标 14：基层医疗卫生机构开展 35 岁以上首诊测血压的情况

1. 来源

早期发现与监测能力模块。

2. 分值

5 分。

3. 指标含义

2011 年，开展 35 岁以上居民首诊测血压的被调查基层医疗卫生机构的比例。

4. 赋值方法

赋值=5×被调查基层医疗卫生机构开展 35 岁以上居民首诊测血压的比例。

5. 各省（自治区、直辖市）得分及排序情况

各省（自治区、直辖市）综合评估指标 14 得分及排序情况见表 2-119。

表 2-119　各省（自治区、直辖市）“基层开展 35 岁以上首诊测血压”指标得分及排序情况

省（市、区）	基层开展 35 岁以上首诊测血压		排序
	比例（%）	得分	
北京	97.7	4.88	10
天津	94.2	4.71	19
河北	93.3	4.66	21
山西	98.8	4.94	6
内蒙古	86.3	4.32	27
辽宁	82.2	4.11	31
吉林	97.2	4.86	13
黑龙江	84.2	4.21	29
上海	98.6	4.93	7
江苏	99.5	4.98	3
浙江	97.0	4.85	14
安徽	100.0	5.00	1
福建	98.9	4.95	5
江西	88.5	4.42	25
山东	98.1	4.91	8
河南	91.9	4.59	22
湖北	98.1	4.91	8
湖南	89.9	4.50	24
广东	99.1	4.96	4
广西	96.8	4.84	15
海南	93.8	4.69	20
重庆	97.7	4.89	10
四川	95.6	4.78	16
贵州	95.0	4.75	18
云南	97.5	4.88	12

续 表

省（市、区）	基层开展 35 岁以上首诊测血压		排序
	比例（%）	得分	
西藏	25.0	1.25	32
陕西	95.4	4.77	17
甘肃	88.3	4.42	26
青海	100.0	5.00	1
宁夏	85.7	4.29	28
新疆	90.0	4.50	23
兵团	83.3	4.17	30

指标 15：开展全民健康生活方式行动的情况

1. 来源

干预与管理能力模块。

2. 分值

5 分。

3. 指标含义

2011 年开展全民健康生活方式行动的县（区）比例。

4. 赋值方法

据《中国慢性病防治工作规划（2012~2015 年）》到 2015 年全民健康生活方式行动覆盖全国 50%的县（市、区）。

省内开展全民健康生活方式行动的县（区）比例≥50%，则赋值 5 分；≥37.5%且<50%，则赋值 4 分；≥25%且<37.5%，则赋值 3 分；≥12.5%且<25%，则赋值 2 分；≥0 且<12.5%，则赋值 1 分；=0%，则赋值 0 分。

5. 各省（自治区、直辖市）得分及排序情况

各省（自治区、直辖市）综合评估指标 15 得分及排序情况见表 2-120。

表 2-120 各省（自治区、直辖市）“开展全民健康生活方式行动”指标得分及排序情况

省（市、区）	开展全民健康生活方式行动		排序
	比例（%）	得分	
北京	72.2	5.00	5
天津	100.0	5.00	1
河北	59.1	5.00	11
山西	57.1	5.00	15

续　表

省（市、区）	开展全民健康生活方式行动		排序
	比例（%）	得分	
内蒙古	27.3	3.00	30
辽宁	47.6	4.00	21
吉林	66.1	5.00	6
黑龙江	52.3	5.00	19
上海	83.3	5.00	3
江苏	65.8	5.00	7
浙江	79.6	5.00	4
安徽	37.8	4.00	26
福建	43.0	4.00	23
江西	47.5	4.00	22
山东	64.5	5.00	8
河南	63.8	5.00	9
湖北	58.6	5.00	12
湖南	35.7	3.00	27
广东	58.3	5.00	13
广西	27.9	3.00	29
海南	60.0	5.00	10
重庆	86.8	5.00	2
四川	41.0	4.00	24
贵州	57.3	5.00	14
云南	14.7	2.00	32
西藏	24.2	2.00	31
陕西	54.6	5.00	17
甘肃	41.0	4.00	25
青海	55.0	5.00	16
宁夏	52.6	5.00	18
新疆	29.8	3.00	28
兵团	47.8	4.00	20

指标 16：基层医疗卫生机构高血压患者血压控制情况

1. 来源

干预与管理能力模块。

2. 分值

5 分。

3. 指标含义

2011 年，被调查基层医疗卫生机构高血压患者血压控制率。

4. 赋值方法

据《中国慢性病防治工作规划（2012~2015 年）》要求到 2015 年管理人群血压、血糖控制率达到 60%。

控制率=2011 年随访 4 次以上患者中最近一次血压达标人数/2011 年管理高血压患者人数×100%。

省内如被调查基层医疗卫生机构高血压患者控制率≥60%，则赋值 5 分；≥45% 且 <60%，则赋值 4 分；≥30% 且<45%，则赋值 3 分；≥15% 且<30%，则赋值 2 分；≥0 且 <15%，则赋值 1 分；=0，则赋值 0 分。

5. 各省（自治区、直辖市）得分及排序情况

各省（自治区、直辖市）综合评估指标 16 得分及排序情况见表 2-121。

表 2-121　各省（自治区、直辖市）“血压控制率”指标得分及排序情况

省（市、区）	血压控制率		排序
	控制率（%）	得分	
北京	59.3	4.00	7
天津	66.1	5.00	3
河北	59.5	4.00	6
山西	54.5	4.00	10
内蒙古	48.3	4.00	22
辽宁	48.5	4.00	21
吉林	52.2	4.00	15
黑龙江	47.8	4.00	23
上海	38.1	3.00	28
江苏	65.0	5.00	4
浙江	57.4	4.00	8
安徽	51.4	4.00	17
福建	36.0	3.00	29
江西	47.8	4.00	23
山东	51.8	4.00	16
河南	51.0	4.00	19
湖北	53.2	4.00	11

续　表

省（市、区）	血压控制率		排序
	控制率（%）	得分	
湖南	51.4	4.00	17
广东	44.2	3.00	26
广西	68.1	5.00	1
海南	45.5	4.00	25
重庆	53.2	4.00	11
四川	64.2	5.00	5
贵州	34.7	3.00	30
云南	43.5	3.00	27
西藏	1.3	1.00	32
陕西	52.4	4.00	14
甘肃	52.7	4.00	13
青海	56.0	4.00	9
宁夏	67.5	5.00	2
新疆	49.2	4.00	20
兵团	16.9	2.00	31

指标 17：基层医疗卫生机构糖尿病患者血糖控制情况

1. 来源

干预与管理能力模块。

2. 分值

5 分。

3. 指标含义

被调查基层医疗卫生机构糖尿病患者血糖控制率。

4. 赋值方法

据《中国慢性病防治工作规划（2012~2015 年）》要求，到 2015 年管理人群血压、血糖控制率达到 60%。

控制率=2011 年随访 4 次以上患者中最近一次血糖达标人数/2011 年管理糖尿病患者人数×100%。

省内被调查基层医疗卫生机构糖尿病患者控制率≥60%，则赋值 5 分；≥45%且<60%，则赋值 4 分；≥30%且<45%，则赋值 3 分；≥15%且<30%，则赋值 2 分；≥0 且<15%，则赋值 1 分；=0，则赋值 0 分。

5. 各省（自治区、直辖市）得分及排序情况各省（自治区、直辖市）综合评估指标 17 得分及排序情况见表 2-122。

表 2-122　各省（自治区、直辖市）“血糖控制率”指标得分及排序情况

省（市、区）	血糖控制率		排序
	控制率（%）	得分	
北京	54.2	4.00	8
天津	67.8	5.00	1
河北	60.2	5.00	5
山西	52.0	4.00	13
内蒙古	54.7	4.00	7
辽宁	50.3	4.00	18
吉林	50.3	4.00	19
黑龙江	50.4	4.00	17
上海	47.1	4.00	22
江苏	64.0	5.00	2
浙江	52.8	4.00	10
安徽	51.1	4.00	16
福建	33.2	3.00	29
江西	53.8	4.00	9
山东	46.9	4.00	23
河南	52.3	4.00	12
湖北	44.6	3.00	25
湖南	51.9	4.00	14
广东	31.5	3.00	30
广西	61.7	5.00	4
海南	49.9	4.00	20
重庆	46.6	4.00	24
四川	63.6	5.00	3
贵州	40.7	3.00	28
云南	43.9	3.00	26
西藏	0.0	0.00	32
陕西	51.5	4.00	15
甘肃	49.7	4.00	21

续　表

省（市、区）	血糖控制率		排序
	控制率（%）	得分	
青海	52.4	4.00	11
宁夏	57.8	4.00	6
新疆	42.6	3.00	27
兵团	15.1	2.00	31

指标 18：基层医疗卫生机构同时开展高血压和糖尿病患者双向转诊的情况

1. 来源

干预与管理能力模块。

2. 分值

5 分。

3. 指标含义

2011 年，同时开展高血压和糖尿病患者双向转诊的被调查基层医疗卫生机构的比例。

4. 赋值方法

赋值 = 5×被调查基层医疗卫生机构同时开展高血压和糖尿病患者双向转诊的比例。

5. 各省（自治区、直辖市）得分及排序情况

各省（自治区、直辖市）综合评估指标 18 得分及排序情况见表 2-123。

表 2-123　各省（自治区、直辖市）“基层同时开展高血压和糖尿病患者双向转诊”指标得分及排序情况

省（市、区）	基层同时开展高血压和糖尿病患者双向转诊		排序
	比例（%）	得分	
北京	50.6	2.53	7
天津	39.1	1.96	21
河北	34.6	1.73	25
山西	36.9	1.85	24
内蒙古	26.3	1.32	30
辽宁	32.7	1.64	26
吉林	31.0	1.55	27
黑龙江	37.8	1.89	22
上海	48.6	2.43	12
江苏	56.5	2.83	3

续 表

省（市、区）	基层同时开展高血压和糖尿病患者双向转诊		排序
	比例（%）	得分	
浙江	47.9	2.39	14
安徽	50.8	2.54	6
福建	49.5	2.47	10
江西	42.3	2.12	19
山东	50.9	2.55	5
河南	43.1	2.15	18
湖北	61.0	3.05	2
湖南	53.5	2.67	4
广东	49.1	2.46	11
广西	48.4	2.42	13
海南	6.3	0.31	31
重庆	43.7	2.18	16
四川	43.6	2.18	17
贵州	27.0	1.35	29
云南	46.9	2.35	15
西藏	0.0	0.00	32
陕西	37.0	1.85	23
甘肃	41.5	2.07	20
青海	50.0	2.50	8
宁夏	28.6	1.43	28
新疆	62.0	3.10	1
兵团	50.0	2.50	9

指标 19：疾控中心参与基层医疗卫生机构考核或评估的情况

1. 来源

评估能力模块。

2. 分值

5 分。省、地市、县（区）三级所占比重分别为 4∶2∶4；直辖市中市级和县（区）两级所占比重分别为 4∶6。

3. 指标含义

2011 年，省、地市和县（区）三级疾控中心参与基层医疗卫生机构考核或评估的比例。

4. 赋值方法

省级赋值，省级参与基层医疗卫生机构考核或评估则赋值 2 分，没有则为 0 分；地市级赋值 = 1×参与基层医疗卫生机构考核或评估的地市级疾控中心比例；县（区）级赋值 = 2×参与基层医疗卫生机构考核或评估的县（区）级疾控中心比例。直辖市因没有地市一级，其赋值情况略有不同，直辖市级赋值与省（自治区）级一致；县（区）级赋值 = 3×本直辖市内参与基层医疗卫生机构考核或评估的县（区）级疾控中心比例。

5. 各省（自治区、直辖市）得分及排序情况

各省（自治区、直辖市）综合评估指标 19 得分及排序情况见表 2-124。

表 2-124 各省（自治区、直辖市）“疾控中心参与基层医疗卫生机构考核或评估”指标得分及排序情况

省（市、区）	省级		地市级		县（区）级		合计得分	排序
	机构	得分	比例（%）	得分	比例（%）	得分		
北京	1	2	—	—	94.4	2.83	4.83	5
天津	1	2	—	—	100.0	3.00	5.00	1
河北	1	2	90.9	0.91	85.8	1.72	4.63	8
山西	1	2	36.4	0.36	74.0	1.48	3.84	18
内蒙古	0	0	66.7	0.67	68.7	1.37	2.04	30
辽宁	1	2	71.4	0.71	61.9	1.24	3.95	16
吉林	0	0	100.0	1.00	83.9	1.68	2.68	24
黑龙江	1	2	84.6	0.85	59.9	1.20	4.04	15
上海	1	2	—	—	100.0	3.00	5.00	1
江苏	1	2	84.6	0.85	95.5	1.91	4.76	6
浙江	1	2	100.0	1.00	94.3	1.89	4.89	4
安徽	1	2	81.3	0.81	93.9	1.88	4.69	7
福建	1	2	55.6	0.56	62.8	1.26	3.81	19
江西	1	2	45.5	0.45	35.4	0.71	3.16	22
山东	0	0	64.7	0.65	75.2	1.50	2.15	28
河南	0	0	58.8	0.59	58.9	1.18	1.77	31
湖北	1	2	76.9	0.77	90.8	1.82	4.59	10
湖南	0	0	71.4	0.71	69.0	1.38	2.09	29
广东	1	2	81.0	0.81	81.6	1.63	4.44	12
广西	1	2	85.7	0.86	69.8	1.40	4.25	13
海南	0	0	50.0	0.50	85.0	1.70	2.20	26
重庆	1	2	—	—	97.4	2.92	4.92	3

续　表

省（市、区）	省级		地市级		县（区）级		合计得分	排序
	机构	得分	比例（%）	得分	比例（%）	得分		
四川	1	2	66.7	0.67	73.2	1.46	4.13	14
贵州	1	2	66.7	0.67	56.2	1.12	3.79	20
云南	1	2	93.8	0.94	83.0	1.66	4.60	9
西藏	0	0	0.0	0.00	9.1	0.18	0.18	32
陕西	0	0	80.0	0.80	87.0	1.74	2.54	25
甘肃	0	0	80.0	0.80	68.7	1.37	2.17	27
青海	1	2	62.5	0.63	62.5	1.25	3.88	17
宁夏	1	2	80.0	0.80	84.2	1.68	4.48	11
新疆	1	2	28.6	0.29	41.5	0.83	3.12	23
兵团	1	2	64.3	0.64	53.7	1.07	3.72	21

指标 20：疾控中心慢性病防控人员人均发表论文的情况

1. 来源

科研能力模块。

2. 分值

5 分。省、地市、县（区）三级所占比重分别为 4∶2∶4；直辖市中市级和县（区）级所占比重分别为 4∶6。

3. 指标含义

2011 年，省、地市和县（区）三级疾控中心慢性病防控在岗人员人均在国内外期刊上以第一作者或通讯作者发表慢性病方面论文的数量。

4. 赋值方法

据《疾控预防控制工作绩效评估标准》要求省级技术人员人均发表论文数量应达到 0.5 篇；地市级技术人员人均发表论文数量应达到 0.3 篇；县（区）级技术人员人均发表论文数量应达到 0.15 篇。省级赋值，人均数量=省级疾控中心在国内外期刊上以第一作者或通讯作者发表慢性病方面中英文论文总数量/省级疾控中心慢性病防控在岗人员数量，人均数量≥0.5 则赋值 2 分、<0.5 则赋值 0 分；地市级赋值，人均数量=地市级疾控中心在国内外期刊上以第一作者或通讯作者发表慢性病方面中英文论文总数量/地市级疾控中心慢性病防控在岗人员数量，人均数量≥0.3 则赋值 1 分、<0.3 则赋值 0 分；县（区）级赋值，人均数量=县（区）疾控中心在国内外期刊上以第一作者或通讯作者发表慢性病方面中英文论文数量/县（区）级疾控慢性病防控在岗人员数量，人均数量≥0.15 则赋值 2 分、<0.15 则赋值 0 分；直辖市因没有地市一级，其赋值情况略有不同，直辖市级赋值与省（自治区）级一致；县（区）级赋值，人均数量≥0.15 则赋值 3 分、<0.15 则赋值 0 分。

5. 各省（自治区、直辖市）得分及排序情况

各省（自治区、直辖市）综合评估指标 20 得分及排序情况见表 2-125。

表 2-125 各省（自治区、直辖市）“疾控中心慢性病防控人员人均发表论文”指标得分及排序情况

省（市、区）	省级		地市级		县（区）级		合计得分	排序
	均数	得分	均数	得分	均数	得分		
北京	0.53	2	—	—	0.12	0.00	2.00	3
天津	0.67	2	—	—	0.11	0.00	2.00	3
河北	0.12	0	0.15	0.00	0.00	0.00	0.00	19
山西	0.00	0	0.00	0.00	0.01	0.00	0.00	19
内蒙古	0.50	2	0.26	0.00	0.00	0.00	2.00	3
辽宁	0.73	2	0.14	0.00	0.00	0.00	2.00	3
吉林	0.00	0	0.20	0.00	0.01	0.00	0.00	19
黑龙江	0.00	0	0.04	0.00	0.00	0.00	0.00	19
上海	0.71	2	—	—	0.42	3.00	5.00	1
江苏	1.00	2	0.52	1.00	0.17	2.00	5.00	1
浙江	0.43	0	0.58	1.00	0.20	2.00	3.00	3
安徽	1.00	2	0.18	0.00	0.05	0.00	2.00	3
福建	0.50	2	0.25	0.00	0.02	0.00	2.00	3
江西	0.75	2	0.14	0.00	0.01	0.00	2.00	3
山东	0.58	2	0.13	0.00	0.08	0.00	2.00	3
河南	0.50	2	0.14	0.00	0.01	0.00	2.00	3
湖北	0.50	2	0.45	1.00	0.02	0.00	3.00	3
湖南	0.25	0	0.10	0.00	0.01	0.00	0.00	19
广东	0.89	2	0.18	0.00	0.08	0.00	2.00	3
广西	0.55	2	0.02	0.00	0.01	0.00	2.00	3
海南	0.33	0	0.00	0.00	0.00	0.00	0.00	19
重庆	0.83	2	—	—	0.01	0.00	2.00	3
四川	0.60	2	0.16	0.00	0.01	0.00	2.00	3
贵州	0.21	0	0.00	0.00	0.00	0.00	0.00	19
云南	0.00	0	0.09	0.00	0.00	0.00	0.00	19
西藏	0.00	0	0.00	0.00	0.00	0.00	0.00	19
陕西	0.00	0	0.02	0.00	0.01	0.00	0.00	19

续 表

省（市、区）	省级		地市级		县（区）级		合计得分	排序
	均数	得分	均数	得分	均数	得分		
甘肃	0.14	0	0.04	0.00	0.02	0.00	0.00	19
青海	0.00	0	0.21	0.00	0.01	0.00	0.00	19
宁夏	0.25	0	0.12	0.00	0.00	0.00	0.00	19
新疆	0.38	0	0.13	0.00	0.00	0.00	0.00	19
兵团	2.00	2	0.00	0.00	0.00	0.00	2.00	3

综合评估结果：将20个指标得分相加算出综合得分，并据此为31个省（自治区、直辖市）和新疆生产建设兵团排序，结果见表2-126。

表2-126　2011年全国慢性病防控能力调查综合评价排序结果

编号	省（自治区、直辖市）	综合得分	综合排序
1	北京	72.46	4
2	天津	74.83	3
3	河北	61.38	8
4	山西	55.67	18
5	内蒙古	47.07	28
6	辽宁	58.05	12
7	吉林	60.27	9
8	黑龙江	53.50	19
9	上海	84.34	1
10	江苏	77.21	2
11	浙江	71.65	5
12	安徽	55.91	17
13	福建	52.66	21
14	江西	51.89	22
15	山东	63.98	7
16	河南	56.60	15
17	湖北	59.21	11
18	湖南	45.32	29
19	广东	59.83	10
20	广西	52.92	20

续　表

编号	省（自治区、直辖市）	综合得分	综合排序
21	海南	49.88	25
22	重庆	65.85	6
23	四川	57.89	13
24	贵州	44.17	30
25	云南	48.64	26
26	西藏	15.65	32
27	陕西	51.74	23
28	甘肃	50.35	24
29	青海	56.41	16
30	宁夏	56.86	14
31	新疆	47.23	27
32	兵团	44.17	31

十一、规划相关基线指标

2012 年 5 月由原卫生部等 15 部门联合制定了《中国慢性病防治工作规划（2012～2015 年）》（以下简称《规划》），《规划》中明确指出，到 2015 年要达到以下具体目标：

——慢性病防控核心信息人群知晓率达 50%以上，35 岁以上成人血压和血糖知晓率分别达到 70%和 50%。

——全民健康生活方式行动覆盖全国 50%的县（市、区），国家级慢性病综合防控示范区覆盖全国 10%以上县（市、区）。

——全国人均每日食盐摄入量下降到 9 克以下；成年人吸烟率降低到 25%以下；经常参加体育锻炼的人数比例达到 32%以上；成人肥胖率控制在 12%以内，儿童青少年不超过 8%。

——高血压和糖尿病患者规范管理率达到 40%，管理人群血压、血糖控制率达到 60%；脑卒中发病率上升幅度控制在 5%以内，死亡率下降 5%。

——30%的癌症高发地区开展重点癌症早诊早治工作。

——40 岁以上慢性阻塞性肺病患病率控制在 8%以内。

——适龄儿童窝沟封闭覆盖率达到 20%以上，12 岁儿童患龋率控制在 25%以内。

——全人群死因监测覆盖全国 90%的县（市、区），慢性病及危险因素监测覆盖全国 50%的县（市、区），营养状况监测覆盖全国 15%的县（市、区）。

——慢性病防控专业人员占各级疾控机构专业人员的比例达 5%以上。

本次调查中共涉及以上 24 个具体指标中的 7 个。分别为高血压和糖尿病患者规范管理率，管理人群血压、血糖控制率，全人群死因监测覆盖率；慢性病危险因素监测覆盖率和慢性病防控专业人员占各级疾控机构专业人员比例。

（一）高血压患者规范管理率

本次调查中高血压患者规范管理率（82.6%）的计算方法是参照国家基本公共卫生服务规范的标准，即高血压患者规范管理率=规范管理高血压患者人数/管理的高血压患者人数×100%。

（二）糖尿病患者规范管理率

本次调查中糖尿病患者规范管理率（82.5%）的计算方法是参照国家基本公共卫生服务规范的标准，即糖尿病患者规范管理率=规范管理糖尿病患者人数/管理的糖尿病患者人数×100%。

（三）管理人群血压控制率

本次调查的基层医疗卫生机构管理人群血压控制率为 53.1%，距《规划》要求相差 6.9 个百分点。2011 年已经达到《规划》中“管理人群血压控制率达到 60%”要求的省（自治区、直辖市）有 5 个，调查中管理人群控制率最高的省份为 68.1%，最低的仅为 1.3%。

（四）管理人群血糖控制率

本次调查的基层医疗卫生机构管理人群血糖控制率为 51.7%，距《规划》要求相差 8.3 个百分点。2011 年已经达到《规划》中“管理人群血糖控制率达到 60%”要求的省（自治区、直辖市）为 5 个，调查中管理人群控制率最高的省份为 67.8%，最低的仅为 0%。

（五）全人群死因监测覆盖率

本次调查显示 2011 年全人群死因监测覆盖全国 54.1%的县（市、区），与《规划》中规定的“全人群死因监测覆盖全国 90%的县（市、区）”的要求还有较大的差距。

（六）慢性病危险因素监测覆盖率

本次调查显示 2011 年除血脂外其他各项慢性病危险因素监测覆盖全国 19.2%的县（市、区），与《规划》中规定的“慢性病及危险因素监测覆盖全国 50%的县（市、区）”的要求还有较大的差距。

（七）慢性病防控专业人员占各级疾控机构专业人员比例

本次调查显示，省、地市、县（区）各级疾控在岗人员分别为 13 006、40 507 和 147 537人。根据《2012 年中国卫生统计年鉴》显示，2011 年省、地市、县（区）技术人员占总人员比例分别为 78.4%，81.3%和 82.1%。据此推算省、地市、县（区）各级疾控专业人员数量分别为 10 197、32 932、121 127 人。

2011 年省级慢性病防控专业人员占各级疾控机构专业人员比例为 3.0%，地市级慢性病防控专业人员占各级疾控机构专业人员比例为 2.7%，县（区）级慢性病防控专业人员占各级疾控机构专业人员比例为 3.4%。各级慢性病防控专业人员占各级疾控机构专业人员比例与《规划》中规定的“慢性病防控专业人员占各级疾控机构专业人员的比例达 5%以上”的要求均有一定差距；2011 年仅有 1 个省份内的地市级疾控已经达到《规划》中指标的要求，地市级比例最高的为 6.7%，最低的仅为 1.2%；2011 年有 4 个省份的县（区）级疾控已经达到《规划》中指标的要求，县（区）级比例最高的为 8.7%，最低的为 0.8%。

43.7%（2009 年和 2008 年分别为 38.2%、34.7%）。省级比例最高，达到 88.6%，地市和县（区）级分别为 64.1%和 37.9%。地区分布来看，东部地区工作人员中以本科学历比重最大，为 45.8%；中部和西部则以大专学历人员为主，比例分别为 41.6%和 44.7%。东部地区省级疾控中心中具有硕士和博士学历的人员比例达 46.9%。地市和县（区）级疾控中心中本科以下学历人员还占有较大比例，特别是中、西部县（区）级疾控中心，本科以下学历人员所占比例均近 70%。这说明我国慢性病防控队伍人员配备并不平衡，经济发展好的东部地区吸引了更多的高学历人才，而中、西部地区，高学历人才较少。

2011 年，我国慢性病防控人员具有医学专业背景的人员比例达 89.9%，且以预防医学（或公共卫生）和临床医学为主要专业，分别占 40.1%和 30.1%。省级疾控中心中慢性病防控人员以预防医学（或公共卫生）背景所占比例最高，为 69.8%，地市和县（区）级这一比例有所下降，分别为 50.4%和 36.9%；但在三级疾控中心中临床医学背景人员的比例呈上升趋势，分别为 12.8%、26.4%和 31.6%，以上趋势与 2009 年调查结果一致。从地区分布来看，东、中、西部具有医学背景人员的比例均较高，分别为 90.50%、86.60%和 92.40%。各地同样呈现出从省、地市再到县（区），预防医学或公共卫生背景人员比例下降，而临床医学背景人员比例上升的趋势。各级疾控中心慢性病防控在岗人员中 77.2%取得执业资格，省、地市和县（区）分别为 85.5%、85.6%和 75.2%，东、中、西部地区该比例分别为 78.6%、73.1 和 79.2%。全国慢性病防控人员仍以具有初级职称的人员比例最高（38.9%），但较 2009 年比例（40.9%）略有下降。省级人员中以具有中级职称的比例最高（37.9%）较 2009 年的调查结果有所变化，2009 年以具有高级职称的比例最高。县（区）级仍以具有初级职称的比例最高（41.7%）较 2009 年的比例（43.5%）有所降低。

对基层医疗卫生机构卫生技术在岗人员的调查发现东、中、西部社区卫生服务中心的卫生技术在岗人员的均数均高于乡镇卫生院，被调查社区卫生服务中心卫生技术在岗人员均数为 49.4 人，乡镇卫生院均数为 30.3 人。其中东部地区的社区卫生服务中心的卫生技术在岗人员均数最高，为 60.1 人，西部乡镇卫生院最少，为 20.7 人。

3. 经费配置

2011 年，全国配置慢性病防控工作经费的疾控中心比例为 57.3%，比 2009 年的比例（40.2%）有所提高。其中省级明显高于全国平均水平高达 96.9%，地市级为 76.0%，县（区）级仅为 54.6%。与 2009 年省、地市和县（区）三级比例（100%、55.7%和 37.4%）相比，除省级有所降低外，地市和县（区）两级均有较大幅度增加。东部地区各级疾控中心经费配置情况均好于中部和西部地区，西部县（区）级配置经费的机构比例最低（48.5%），但已较 2009 年（仅 26.2%）有大幅增长。

2011 年，不同级别和地区疾控中心经费配备数额相差悬殊，省级疾控中心平均经费为 181.6 万元，中位数为 80 万元，东部地区某省经费最高达 1329.8 万元，中部地区某省经费最低（仅 30.5 万元），但相比 2009 年调查时西部某省 1.7 万元的最低值已有较大提高。地市级和县（区）级疾控中心平均工作经费分别为 17.0 万元和 13.7 万元，中位数分别为 5 万元和 4.7 万元。其中工作经费最少的仅 1000 元。从地区分布来看，东部地区的平均工作经费和中位数都要高于中、西部地区。

2011 年，全国各级疾控中心的慢性病防控工作经费占疾控中心业务经费比例为 4.4%，较 2009 年（2.7%）有所增长。省、地市、县（区）分别为 2.0%、3.1%和 7.4%，2009 年，三级的比例分别为 2.8%、2.2%和 2.9%，地市和县（区）的比例均有较大幅度提高，县（区）级比例增长近 2.5 倍。从地区分布来看，东部地区的省级和地市级疾控中心慢性病防控工作经费占疾控中心业务经费的比例均高于中、西部地区，而县（区）级这一比例则以西部地区最高（7.9%）。

基层医疗卫生机构的经费情况：2011 年是深化医药卫生体制改革开展基本公共卫生服务均等化的第 3 年，95.5%的被调查机构获得了基本公共卫生服务经费，较 2009 年（74.3%）有较大增长。基层医疗卫生机构获得财政拨款的平均数额为 85.4 万元，社区卫生服务中心和乡镇卫生院分别为 117.9 万元和 52.4 万元。东、中、西部地区基本公共卫生服务经费的平均数额分别为 128.3 万元、63.6 万元和 53.9 万元，中、西部较东部有较大差距。被调查基层医疗卫生机构 34.8%的财政拨款来源于基本公共卫生服务项目，社区卫生服务中心和乡镇卫生院的这一比例分别为 34.1%和 36.3%，差异不大。从地区分布来看，中部（42.4%）高于东、西部（分别为 31.8%和 37.9%）。这也说明执行基本公共卫生服务工作在基层医疗机构日常工作中的比重较大。

4. 设备配置

基层医疗卫生机构配置慢性病防控相关设备的情况能在一定程度上反映其提供慢性病防控服务的能力。本次调查发现，基层医疗卫生机构配备基本诊疗设备如体重秤、身高计、腰围尺、血压计、血糖仪的比例均在 90%以上，心电图机、B 超、生化仪、健教设备和 X 线机的配备比例分别为 82.8%、79.5%、72.1%、71.9%和 66.8%。肺功能检测工作相对专业性较强，肺功能仪的配备比例也最低，仅为 16.3%。在被调查基层医疗卫生机构中，乡镇卫生院配备各类慢性病防控相关设备的比例与 2009 年相比，已有大幅度增加，但除 X 线机外，仍低于社区卫生服务中心的各项设备配备比例。

尽管基层配备各项设备的比例已较 2009 年调查时有所提高，但由于国家基本公共卫生服务项目需要在所有基层医疗卫生机构开展，缺乏相关设备将无法保障各项健康管理服务工作的顺利开展。

（三）教育培训与指导能力

慢性病防控教育培训和指导能力是各级慢性病防控机构的重要防控能力之一。本次调查了各地、各级疾控中心及基层医疗卫生机构的培训能力、指导能力和知识普及能力等方面的信息。

调查发现，不同级别疾控中心开展培训和参加培训的能力还存在一定差距，省级疾控中心开展和参加培训的能力高于地市和县（区）级，但地市和县（区）级疾控中心开展和参加培训的情况较 2009 年有较大程度提高。在指导能力方面，从开展指导的机构比例来看，西部地区和县（区）级疾控中心能力偏低。基层医疗卫生机构开展对社区卫生服务站和村卫生室的技术指导工作情况与 2009 年相比有大幅度提高。在知识普及能力方面，各地均有一定比例的基层医疗卫生机构会在健康宣传日期间开展相关知识宣传活动，但是各类宣传活动的普及性还存在一定的差异。

1. 培训能力

2011 年全国各级疾控中心举办过慢性病相关培训的比例为 67. 2%，比 2009 年的 43. 5% 上升了 23. 7 个百分点；省、地市、县（区）级疾控中心举办慢性病相关培训的比例分别为 100. 0%、70. 5%、66. 4%，比 2009 年分别上升了 3. 1、20. 2 和 24. 3 个百分点。从类别来看，举办国际级和国家级慢性病培训的比例偏低。从开展培训的级别来看，各级疾控中心均以开展本级培训的比例最高。2011 年被调查基层医疗卫生机构中开展培训的比例为 82. 5%，较 2009 年的比例（58. 8%）有较大幅度的提高，主要是乡镇卫生院开展培训比例提高较大的结果（2011 年 83. 8%，2009 年为 44. 6%）。

2011 年全国各级疾控中心派人员参加慢性防控相关培训的比例为 78. 5%，比 2009 年的 53. 8%上升了 24. 7 个百分点。派人员参加培训的机构比例从地区分布和级别来看，与 2009 年相同，均呈现东、中、西部和省、地市、县（区）依次下降的趋势，西部和县（区）级疾控中心派人员参加相关培训的比例最低，人员培训工作有待进一步加强。与 2009 年相比，2011 年省级疾控中心派人员参加培训的比例下降了 3. 1 个百分点，主要原因在于西部地区只有 84. 6%的省级疾控中心派人员参加了培训（2009 年为 92. 3%），而东、中部地区省级均达到 100. 0%。2011 年县（区）级疾控中心派人员参加省和地市级疾控中心培训的比例分别为 50. 9%、54. 2%，比 2009 年分别上升了 23. 1 和 22. 6 个百分点，但作为慢性病防控的具体实施单位，县（区）级疾控中心派人员参加相关培训的比例仍然偏低。被调查基层医疗卫生机构中派人员参加慢性病防控相关培训的比例为 89. 7%，比 2009 年上升了 21. 4 个百分点。

调查发现，2011 年各级疾控中心对各项技能培训的需求均较高，其中需求最高的是高危人群管理相关技能，比例为 92. 6%；最低的是死因监测技能，比例为 86. 9%。应根据各级疾控中心具体需求情况开展有针对性的培训才能达到事半功倍的效果。

2. 技术指导能力

2011 年地市级疾控中心指导县（区）级疾控中心的比例（85. 5%）和县（区）级疾控中心指导基层医疗卫生机构的比例（79. 5%）均较 2009 年（分别为 64. 7%和 48. 3%）有较大幅度提高。对辖区内的社区卫生服务站/村卫生室开展慢性病现场技术指导的被调查基层医疗卫生机构的比例也有所提高（2011 年为 73. 1%，2009 年为 49. 0%）。可见 2011 年，各级单位对慢性病防控工作的重视程度有所提高，同时通过上级机构的有效指导基层机构的慢性病防控工作也将更好的开展。

3. 知识普及能力

2011 年，全国各地基层医疗卫生机构在高血压日、无烟日、糖尿病日开展宣传活动的比例较高，分别为 91.0%、88.5%和 87.8%，而在脑卒中日、心脏病日开展宣传活动的比例均不到 50.0%。基层医疗卫生机构是慢性病防控工作的基底，其开展慢性病防控相关宣传工作，将对慢性病防控相关知识的普及起到十分重要的作用。调查发现，乡镇卫生院开展相关各项活动的比例均低于社区卫生服务中心，可见乡镇卫生院知识普及的能力低于社区卫生服务中心。

（四）合作能力

慢性病防控领域中重要策略之一是发展多部门合作。总体来看，2011 年各级疾控中心与其他部门在慢性病防控方面的合作程度比 2009 年有所提高，但比例仍不高，特别是县（区）级疾控中心与其他机构开展合作的比例较低。

1. 2011 年，与各类机构的合作比例均较 2009 年有所提高。与媒体合作比例 2009 年为 20.2%，2011 年为 36.2%；与医院合作比例 2009 年为 19.7%，2011 年为 28.2%；与专业防办合作比例 2009 年为 4.3%，2011 年 6.1%；与 NGO 合作比例 2009 年为 1.7%，2011 年为 5.9%。

2. 2011 年，在慢性病防控工作中，主要合作机构仍然是媒体和二级及以上医院，合作比例明显高于其他机构。与媒体合作是开展慢性病防控工作最重要的途径之一，媒体宣传，对慢性病防控的政策倡导、健康知识和相关信息的传播起着不可替代的作用。与 2009 年相比，2011 年各级疾控中心与媒体合作的比例有所上升，主要是地市级（2009 年为 38.4%，2011 年为 58.1%）和县（区）级（2009 年为 17.2%，2011 年为 33.2%）有较大幅度的提升。疾控中心和医院都是慢性病防治网络中的重要组成机构，疾控中心与医院开展合作，有助于促进慢性病领域的医防整合，加强慢性病防治工作。2011 年，疾控中心与二级以上医院的合作比例较 2009 年有所提升，也主要是因为地市级（2009 年为 25.7%，2011 年为 36.1%）和县（区）级（2009 年为 19.7%，2011 年为 26.8%）有一定幅度的提升。

3. 2011 年各级疾控中心与各类慢性病防控机构的合作比例均呈现省、地市、县（区）和东、中、西部下降趋势，与 2009 年的趋势一致。

（五）参与能力

1. 疾控中心

2011 年各级疾控中心参与本级卫生行政部门政策制定的比例为 29.6%（2009 年为 13.5%），参与本级卫生以外其他行政部门慢性病防控工作的比例为 30.5%（2009 年为

15.5%），参与上级卫生行政部门或业务机构慢性病防控工作的比例为 19.6%（2009 年为 9.4%）。

疾控中心参与本级卫生行政部门政策制定、本级卫生以外其他行政部门慢性病防控工作、上级卫生行政部门或业务机构慢性病防控工作的比例均呈省、地市、县（区）三级递减，且省级与地市级、县（区）级的差距较大，可见地市级和县（区）级疾控中心慢性病防控参与能力还明显不足。从地区分布来看，东部均高于中部和西部。

2. 基层医疗卫生机构

基层医疗卫生机构参与各级慢性病防控相关项目或科研工作的比例为 12.4%，社区卫生服务中心高于乡镇卫生院。乡镇卫生院参与省级和地市级慢性病防控相关项目或科研工作的比例均还不到 2%。社区卫生服务中心参与各级慢性病防控相关项目或科研工作的比例，其中参与国家级的比例最高（7.6%），参与省级的比例最低（4.3%）；乡镇卫生院参与县（区）级慢性病防控相关项目或科研工作的比例最高（4.1%），参与地市级慢性病防控相关项目或科研工作的比例最低（0.9%）。

东部地区的社区卫生服务中心参与各级慢性病防控相关项目或科研工作的比例均高于中、西部地区；但是东部地区的乡镇卫生院参与各级慢性病防控相关项目或科研工作的比例均低于中部、西部。

（六）慢性病防控监测能力

开展慢性病监测与调查是动态掌握慢性病发病、患病、死亡及危险因素的流行状况和变化趋势，确定慢性病预防控制优先领域，制订政策和评价干预措施效果的重要基础。目前，全国慢性病监测工作主要由各级疾病预防控制中心和部分医疗卫生机构承担，以常规监测和专题调查为主，包括死因监测、慢性病危险因素监测、发病和患病登记等。

1. 各类慢性病相关监测的开展比例整体偏低，特别是基层机构的监测水平亟待提高。

2011 年，各类慢性病监测中，死因监测的开展比例最高（66.1%）与 2009 年开展的比例基本一致（66.3%）。基层医疗机构开展死亡病例报告的比例（57.6%）高于 2009 年（44.8%）。

2011 年，疾控中心开展各类慢性病危险因素监测的比例均较 2009 年有所提高，其中开展血压监测的比例最高，但也仅为 37.1%。可见，慢性病危险因素监测开展水平整体偏低。除血脂监测外，省级开展各类慢性病危险因素监测的比例均在 90%以上，可见慢性病危险因素监测工作已纳入大部分省级疾控中心的常规工作。各类危险因素监测的开展比例均呈现省、地市、县（区）下降趋势，地市和县（区）级疾控中心开展各类慢性病危险因素监测的比例远低于省级。在开展的各类危险因素监测中，均以任务来自于上级机构的比例最高，来自于本级机构的比例其次，来自于国际级的最低。

各级疾控中心开展慢性病发病与患病报告的比例较 2009 年有所上升，其中开展恶性肿瘤登记报告的比例为35.5%，目前恶性肿瘤登记已纳入中央转移支付地方重大公共卫生项目并作为慢性病综合防控示范区的考核指标之一，推动了此项工作的开展。脑卒中与心肌梗死病例报告的开展比例相对较低，分别为22.3%和21.1%，但均较2009年有所上升。基层医疗卫生机构是我国开展慢性病发病患病报告的主要机构，调查发现2011年基层医疗卫生机构开展脑卒中与心肌梗死病例报告工作的比例分别为27.1%和23.8%，较2009年(18.6%和13.0%）均有所提高，但仍处于较低的水平。

2. 在开展的各类慢性病相关监测中，地区代表性较好，其中覆盖所有县（区）/街道和乡镇的比例均在50%以上，数据能更好地反映被监测地区的实际情况。

开展的各类监测中覆盖所有县（区）/街道和乡镇或虽没有覆盖所有县（区）/街道和乡镇但具有当地代表性的比例分别为：死因监测90.0%、烟草使用监测88.5%、膳食监测88.5%、身体活动监测87.7%、酒精使用监测80.6%、超重肥胖监测87.9%、血压监测90.8%、血糖监测90.1%、血脂监测86.9%。恶性肿瘤报告91.9%、脑卒中报告93.5%、心肌梗死报告94.0%。目前开展的各类监测中，数据具有较好的代表性，能为制定当地慢性病防控工作规划、计划与实施慢性病综合防控措施提供客观的依据，但目前慢性病相关监测的地区覆盖度仍需提高。

3. 2011年，在开展的各类慢性病相关监测中，编写年报仍然是信息发布及利用的主要形式。

目前，慢性病相关监测的信息主要集中在专业领域发布或利用，形式主要有编写年报和发表论文等，而真正能扩大监测数据影响范围的媒体发布和出版报告等方式利用率较低，这大大降低了监测数据的影响力。

2011年，在开展的各类慢性病相关监测中，监测数据信息发布被采纳的比例均低于70%，其中最低的为死因监测的比例仅为54.8%，最高的为身体活动监测比例为68.6%。开展监测工作的最终目的应该是数据能得到更好地利用，为当地或国家制定慢性病防控政策提供依据，所以提高已开展监测数据的采纳程度与扩大监测工作的覆盖范围同样是当前开展慢性病防控工作的重要任务。

（七）慢性病干预与管理能力

慢性病干预主要面向一般人群、高危人群和患病人群三类，需要疾控中心、基层医疗卫生机构、医院和专业防治机构的密切协作，需要卫生系统外其他部门或单位的支持，需要社会和民众的积极参与。

1. 2011年，各级疾控中心开展主要慢性病及其危险因素干预工作的比例较2009年有所提高，但整体水平仍然较低。

调查显示，2011年，在慢性病患者干预中，排在前两位的是高血压和糖尿病的干预工作，各级疾控中心开展或参与的比例分别为64.1%和62.8%，较2009年分别提高了28.0

和 30.6 个百分点。2011 年其他几种慢性病患者干预工作的开展比例均低于 30%，但比 2009 年分别提高了 2.2~5.3 个百分点。说明随着高血压和糖尿病患者管理纳入基本公共卫生服务项目，这两项工作也成为各级疾控中心开展或参与程度最高的慢性病干预工作。在确保这两项重点工作的同时，其他慢性病患者干预工作较 2009 年也有所提高。开展或参与慢性病高危人群干预的疾控中心的比例为 28.1%，高于 2009 年的调查结果（13.7%）。高血压、糖尿病、恶性肿瘤、脑卒中患者干预工作均以省级疾控中心开展或参与的比例最高，但冠心病和慢性呼吸系统疾病患者干预工作则以县（区）级疾控中心开展或参与的比例最高且呈现县（区）、地市、省级递减趋势。开展或参与高血压、糖尿病、恶性肿瘤、脑卒中和冠心病患者干预工作的比例均呈现东部、西部、中部递减趋势，开展或参与慢性呼吸系统疾病患者干预工作的比例以西部最高、中部次之、东部最低。

慢性病相关危险因素的干预工作中，各级疾控中心开展全民健康生活方式行动的比例最高（52.2%），其中省级高达 93.8%，但仍有两省报告还未开展此项工作。烟草干预工作居第二位，比例为 35.2%。本次调查发现，除全民健康生活方式行动和烟草干预外，开展慢性病相关危险因素干预工作的省级疾控中心的比例均较 2009 年有较大幅下降，地市级变化不大，县（区）级上升较为明显，说明该项工作重心已出现下移趋势，基层参与程度有所提高。

2. 35 岁以上居民首诊测血压和 65 岁以上老年人免费健康体检制度在基层医疗卫生机构中已初步建立，乡镇卫生院早期发现能力与 2009 年相比有大幅度提高。

基层医疗卫生机构是早期发现慢性病患者和高危人群并提供早诊早治的主要机构。2009 年，国家基本公共卫生服务规范将 35 岁以上居民首诊测血压和 65 岁以上老年人健康管理纳入基层医疗卫生机构的常规工作。调查结果显示，2011 年，社区卫生服务中心开展 35 岁以上居民首诊测血压工作的比例为 96.5%，开展 65 岁以上老年人免费健康体检的比例为 90.9%，均较 2009 年的调查结果有一定程度提高（2009 年分别为 89.1% 和 74.8%）。2011 年乡镇卫生院开展这两项工作的比例有很大程度的提高，分别达到 91.7% 和 93.4%，比 2009 年分别上升 47.9 和 48.4 个百分点。可见，2009 年基本公共卫生服务项目刚开展之时，这两项工作呈现在社区卫生服务中心开展较多而在乡镇卫生院开展比例较低的情况，到 2011 年 35 岁以上居民首诊测血压和 65 岁以上老年人免费健康体检制度已在基层医疗卫生机构中初步建立。

在开展 65 岁以上老年人免费健康体检的基层医疗卫生机构中，身高、体重、腰围、血压与血糖测量等这些成本低、易操作的检查项目，开展比例均高于 90%。而血脂、X 线与心电图检查这些成本高、技术性较强的检查项目开展比例较低，尤其是在西部地区和乡镇卫生院，开展情况明显不如东部、中部地区和社区卫生中心。可见，2011 年，乡镇卫生院开展 65 岁以上老年人免费健康体检的比例略高于社区卫生服务中心，但社区卫生服务中心在提供服务项目数量上明显优于乡镇卫生院。

3. 基层医疗卫生机构承担高血压、糖尿病患者管理工作的比例较2009年有较大幅度的提高，辖区管理率也有提高，但相对于庞大的患者人群仍显不足，规范化管理过程和管理效果仍需提高。高危人群管理工作较2009年有一定程度改善，但仍处于较低水平。

2009年，高血压、糖尿病患者管理工作纳入国家基本公共卫生服务项目，并由财政经费给予支持，基层医疗卫生机构是高血压、糖尿病患者管理的主要执行机构。通过两年的发展，2011年调查显示，已有95%左右的基层医疗卫生机构承担了高血压、糖尿病患者建档和管理工作，比例明显高于2009年。管理率、规范管理率和控制率也有不同程度的提高，但水平仍然较低，特别是管理率，据估算，被调查基层医疗卫生机构高血压患者管理率仅为14.2%，糖尿病管理率仅为10.1%。可见，高血压和糖尿病患者管理工作虽已在基层医疗卫生机构普遍开展，但实际受益的人群仅占高血压和糖尿病患者的很少一部分，如何让更多的高血压和糖尿病患者得到社区服务，切实通过社区管理使患者的血压和血糖得到控制，进一步降低高血压和糖尿病的患病率是此项工作的重点。

血压正常高值者和空腹血糖受损/糖耐量减低者是高血压和糖尿病的高危人群，这两类人群如果得不到及时控制，很可能发展成为高血压和糖尿病患者。2011年，基层医疗卫生机构开展血压正常高值者建档工作和糖尿病高危人群即空腹血糖受损/糖耐量减低者建档工作的比例虽较2009年有所提高，但仍处于较低的水平。

（八）慢性病防控评估能力

2011年地市和县（区）级疾控中心或卫生行政部门对本辖区慢性病应对情况的评估能力较2009年有所加强。全国30.6%的卫生行政部门或疾控中心对本辖区慢性病应对情况进行了定期的评估，高于2009年的比例（13.3%）。

2011年调查发现，各级疾控中心参与本辖区基层医疗卫生机构考核评估的比例较高，超过了70%，较2009年的比例明显提高，省、地市、县（区）各级均有不同程度的提高，体现各级疾控中心在基本公共卫生服务工作中发挥了应有的作用。

（九）慢性病科研能力

省级疾控中心相对具有较强的慢性病科研能力，明显高于地市和县（区）级疾控中心；东部地区疾控中心的科研能力高于中、西部地区。但从全国总体水平来看，全国疾控中心慢性病防控方面的科研能力仍然较为薄弱，承担国内和国际科研项目的机构比例仅为6.7%和1.1%（2009年分别为6.1%和3.8%）。2011年，各级疾控中心在国内外发表慢性病方面论文、出版慢性病方面专著及获得科技进步奖的机构比例均较2009年有所下降。全国各级疾控慢性病防控科研能力偏低，有待提高。

二、建议

（一）加强政策倡导，均衡区域发展

2012 年 5 月，国家卫生计生委（原卫生部）等 15 部委联合印发《中国慢性病防治工作规划（2012~2015 年）》（以下简称慢病规划），是我国第一个国家级慢性病综合防治规划，是慢性病防治历程中的“里程碑”。慢病规划指出“各地要围绕规划总体目标和重点工作，结合实际，制订本地防治规划和年度工作计划，认真研究推进规划目标实现的政策和措施，切实解决防治工作中的问题和困难，落实政策保障、人员配备、资金投入、监督奖励等措施，大力加强社会动员，努力形成政府社会防治工作合力”。慢病规划下发后，各省按照慢病规划要求制订本省慢性病防治规划，截至 2013 年底，全国有 19 个省印发或转发省级慢性病防治工作规划，东部 11 省有 6 省下发，中部 8 省有 5 省下发，西部 12 省有 8 省下发，包括，上海、四川、广西、青海、吉林、湖南、河北、山东、河南、云南、安徽、江西、陕西、浙江、内蒙古、海南、广东、贵州、重庆。是否下发省级慢性病规划能够在一定程度上反映本省对慢性病防控工作的重视程度，省级慢性病规划对各省结合当地实际情况有重点地开展防控工作至关重要。对于地市级和县（区）级能够制订可操作可评估的年度实施方案和工作计划则具实际意义。从本次调查结果看，仅有 30.6%和 25.6%的地市和县（区）制订了工作（实施）方案，说明大部分地市和县（区）对于年度工作缺乏合理的考虑和安排。慢病规划中的目标和措施需要各地贯彻和落实，各地应结合当地实际情况制订出具体可行的年度工作方案或工作计划，才能保障慢病规划的有效实施。

在相关政策制定完成后，需要通过多种形式开展政策参与和倡导工作，如邀请政府领导参与慢性病防控活动，通过提交提案或议案等方式是开发领导、争取重视、与其他部门交流、将健康融入公共政策的重要策略和有效途径。本次调查结果显示，上述两方面与 2009 年比较，没有大的改观，均处于较低水平，表明在开发领导、政策倡导方面的能力比较欠缺。特别是在基层，政府对慢性病防控的重视程度较低。

（二）稳步提升慢性病防控基础配置

合理的基础配置是开展慢性病防控工作的基础。基础配置包括人力资源、经费投入和设备配置等方面。慢病规划在目标中明确提出到 2015 年，慢性病防控专业人员占各级疾控中心专业人员的比例达 5%以上。与 2009 年相比，各级疾控中心在慢性病防控专业科室设置和人员配置方面都有稳步的提升。全国慢性病防控在岗人员占疾控中心总在岗人数比例为 4.6%，这与慢病规划中提出的占疾控中心专业人员的比例的指标，在统计上有一定区别。如果按专业人员数进行统计，这一比例会有所降低。根据慢性病规划要求，中国疾控中心也尝试提出具体细化的人力资源配置目标，即到 2015 年，省、地、县（区）三级疾控

中心建立专门的慢性病防控科（所），省级疾控中心慢性病专业人员占中心专业人员的比例达5%以上，地市级达8%以上，县（区）级达10%以上。以这一标准衡量，各地还存在很大的差距。2011年，省、地市、县（区）三级慢性病防控在岗人员占疾控中心总在岗人员比例分别为2.7%、3.4%和5.1%。建议省级和地市级疾控中心设立独立、专门的慢性病防控科所，县（区）级疾控中心保证至少有专职的人员开展慢性病防控常规工作，并明确慢性病专业人员占疾控中心专业人员的比例，保证慢性病防控队伍的持续发展。

从事慢性病防控人员的年龄和就职年数与上次调查无明显变化，仍以中青年为主。特别是西部地区更为年轻化。同时，人员配置在地区间的发展非常不平衡，中西部地区缺乏高素质的工作人员。提示应加大中西部地区的人才引进，相关部门应给予相应的人才引进政策，吸引更多的优秀慢性病防控人才到中西部就业。

在经费投入方面，可以看到，地市级与县（区）级工作经费投入有较大幅度的增加。但不同地区，不同级别疾控中心慢性病防控投入的差别悬殊。过低的工作经费很难保证慢性病防控常规工作的开展。建议各级疾控机构按照慢病规划和慢性病防控工作规范要求，认真梳理常规工作任务，合理编制工作预算，并积极争取常规工作经费，设立相应财政预算。

基础设备配备是基层医疗卫生机构提供服务的基本保障，也是更好的落实医改基本公共卫生服务项目的重要保障，应给予足够的重视。但从目前的调查结果来看，乡镇卫生院与社区卫生服务中心在基础配备情况上存在一定差距，基层医疗卫生机构的配备情况还不能充分满足开展国家基本公共卫生服务工作的需要。国家基本公共卫生服务工作经费已经成为基层医疗卫生机构的主要经费来源之一。在国家基本公共卫生服务人均补偿费用逐年增长的情况下，建议有条件的基层医疗卫生机构探索开展慢性病高危人群管理，并合理安排相应的工作经费。基层医疗卫生机构中基本服务设备的配备情况，社区卫生服务中心明显好于乡镇卫生院，应根据服务需求加强乡镇卫生院的基本设备配备，保障基本服务项目的开展。

（三）发挥省级技术培训和指导能力优势，提高基层慢性病防治的工作能力

在加强各级慢性病防控队伍能力建设方面，应强调和强化逐级技术培训与工作指导相结合的方式。2011年，全国各类培训班参加人次数明显提高，为2009年的近2倍。说明两年间，各级加大了人员培训的力度。从分类看，能够参加国际和国家级培训的人员比例偏低。国家应根据工作任务安排和能力建设需要，多举办高级别高技术水平的能力培训班，着力培养各省级的业务骨干，培养高水平的省级技术力量，开展逐级能力培训。同时在培训内容的设置方面，应结合慢病规划提出的重点工作和慢病工作规范中提出的常规工作设计安排相关内容，针对基层重点培训开展常规工作需要的知识和技能。

结合日常慢性病防控工作，由上级机构对下级机构进行指导是能力建设的重要方法

和手段。调查发现各级疾控中心的现场工作指导落实不到位，接受现场指导的比例不足60%。而对于基层医疗机构的指导工作情况更不理想，特别是西部地区，未能将对基层医疗卫生机构的指导纳入常规工作任务。2012 年 6 月，原卫生部下发了《卫生部关于疾病预防控制机构指导基层开展基本公共卫生服务的意见》，提出各级疾病预防控制机构及相关专业防治机构，特别是县（区）级疾病预防控制机构及相关专业防治机构要以服务基层为宗旨，坚持预防为主、防治结合，指导基层医疗卫生机构切实发挥基本医疗和公共卫生服务的双重网底作用。县（区）级疾控机构应切实提高自身业务能力，发挥好对于基层卫生服务机构的指导职能。

工作既是一个衡量指导机构能力的重要指标，又是一个能有效提高被指导机构慢性病防控能力的手段。调查发现目前地市级疾控中心缺乏对县（区）级疾控中心的指导，在今后的工作中应逐步提高地市级疾控中心的指导能力，充分发挥其应有的作用。深化医药卫生体制改革重新赋予了基层医疗卫生机构承担公共卫生服务工作的职能，因此县（区）级疾控中心应在此方面给予基层医疗卫生机构更多的指导，切实提高基层医疗卫生机构慢性病防控工作能力。

（四）加强多部门的合作，提高慢性病防控决策参与能力

多部门合作共同应对慢性病是重要的慢性病防控策略之一。慢病规划中也明确提出“加强部门间协调沟通，建立慢性病防治工作部际联席会议制度，健全分工明确、各负其责、有效监督的工作机制，协调解决慢性病防治工作重大问题，落实各项防治措施”，并界定了相关部门的职责与任务分工。从调查结果看，目前开展合作比较多的部门，是与媒体部门联合开展慢性病防控宣传工作，而与其他部门的合作则鲜有见到。从国家层面到县（区）层面，多部门合作是慢性病防控中的短板，一直没有突破。从国家层面，应建立由参与慢病规划制订和下发的十五个部委组织的部际联席会议制度。各地也应在各级政府的统一领导下，成立由多部门参与的慢性病防控工作领导小组，明确各部门的职责，分工协作，共同做好慢性病防控工作。

（五）抓好慢性病防控基础性工作，确保工作质量

慢性病监测、综合防治工作是慢性病防控的常规工作和重点工作。目前死因监测工作是开展最广，覆盖面最大的监测工作。66.1%的疾控中心已经开展相关工作。慢病规划中提出“到 2015 年，全人群死因监测覆盖全国 90%的县（市、区），慢性病及危险因素监测覆盖全国 50%的县（市、区），营养状况监测覆盖全国 15%的县（市、区）”的目标。在实现全人群死因监测目标的同时，重点在于提升各监测点的工作质量，报告符合质量要求的数据。对于慢性病及危险因素监测、营养状况调查，由于监测的内容、指标的设定和结果发布方面存在很大的重复性，在一定程度上造成了资源的浪费和加重了基层的工作负担。

应在国家层面进行重新设计、整合和部署，注重省级代表性。对比世界卫生组织发布的《全球非传染性疾病预防和控制综合监测框架》要求，我国在心脑血管事件发病报告方面还存在着差距。首先，慢性病相关监测与报告工作，并不像传染病报告有相关的法律作为保障，特别是心脑血管事件发病报告需要医疗机构的合作。因此，到目前为止，没有国家的报告系统，仅有部分工作基础比较好的发达省份开展了报告工作。国家想启动和开展全国性的报告工作，首先在制度上应给予保障，由卫生计生部门，特别是医院管理部门下发开展此项工作的文件作为依据。同时，应加大对新型信息技术的开发与应用，避免采用传统的手工填报的方式，而是利用信息技术实现现有发病信息的交换，减轻基层医务人员的工作压力和负担。

慢性病综合干预工作要面向一般人群、高风险人群和患者人群。针对全人群开展的全民健康生活方式行动已完成2015年覆盖全国50%的县（区）的既定目标。而工作中存在的问题是在各地启动行动后，如何开展深入、有效果的工作，通过政策倡导、环境建设、技术支持、健康教育和健康促进活动的开展，营造健康生活方式支持环境，促进全民健康生活方式培养，降低人群慢性病危险因素水平，预防慢性病的发生和发展。国家在方案制定和效果评价方面应制定更加严格和细致的标准，各地也不能仅停留在行动启动和健康宣传的层面开展面上的活动。高风险人群的识别和管理工作，一直缺乏明确的项目支撑，全国开展此类工作的机构比例也不多。从国家层面应积极研究相关的技术，开发工作规范与指南，指导各地逐步开展相关工作。各地总结先期试点的工作经验，形成可推广的适宜技术。《国家基本公共卫生服务规范》中65岁以上老年人免费体检制度在基层公共卫生服务机构中落实的比较到位，执行率均值90%以上。高血压和糖尿病患者管理工作的相关执行情况指标变化并不明显。管理率、规范管理率和控制率与2009年相比，提高不明显。能够纳入管理的高血压和糖尿病患者数量明显偏低。如何最大程度的发现社区中的高血压和糖尿病患者成为此项工作的瓶颈。目前存在发现途径较为单一的问题，除了主动上门就诊的病人外，应通过各类机会性筛查，体检和功能社区合作等方式发现和管理患者。

（六）提高各级疾控中心对慢性病应对情况的评估能力，积极开展科学合作

各级疾控中心拥有最完整和最新的慢性病流行情况、防控效果、工作开展情况的数据和资料，这是定期开展区域评估工作的重要基础，也是各级疾控中心的重要职责任务。要充分重视现有监测数据，开展深入分析、利用和数据发布，使疾控系统的监测数据成为各级各地慢性病防控情况的权威数据来源。同时，要扩大监测数据的利用，与社会、经济、环境等数据联合开展数据分析，评价防控工作取得的效果。以真实、客观、权威的分析结果作为当地政策制订、调整和资源优化配置与投入的指挥棒。

各级疾控中心应重视科研能力的提升，以科研工作带动慢性病防控工作。全国慢性病防控队伍人员年轻、学历高、具有做好慢性病科研工作的基本素质。各地应与科技等部门

积极联系，寻求支持，开展慢性病防控适宜技术的研发与应用，提高慢性病防治的科技支撑能力。加强慢性病防治研究和转化基地建设，开发健康教育与健康促进工具，加强科研成果转化和利用，推广慢性病预防、早诊早治早康和规范治疗等适宜技术。加强国内外交流与合作，积极参与慢性病防治全球行动，与国际组织、学术研究机构和院校在人员培训、技术合作和科学研究等方面开展广泛协作。

附　　录

术　　语

1. 疾病预防控制机构：简称疾控机构（疾控中心），本调查中指国家、省（自治区、直辖市）、地（辖区市）、县（区）级疾病预防控制中心和未更名的卫生防疫站。

2. 基层医疗卫生机构：本调查中指社区卫生服务中心和乡镇卫生院。

3. 东、中、西部地区：按《2012 年中国卫生统计年鉴》中的划分标准进行划分。

东部地区包括北京、天津、河北、辽宁、上海、江苏、浙江、福建、山东、广东、海南 11 个省、直辖市；中部地区包括山西、吉林、黑龙江、安徽、江西、河南、湖北、湖南 8 个省；西部地区包括内蒙古、重庆、广西、四川、贵州、云南、西藏、陕西、甘肃、青海、宁夏、新疆 12 个省、自治区、直辖市，新疆生产建设兵团。

4. 慢性病：本次调查中指心脑血管疾病、恶性肿瘤、糖尿病和慢性呼吸系统疾病（不包括精神卫生和口腔）。

5. 慢性病危险因素：本次调查中指不合理饮食、身体活动不足、酒精使用、烟草使用、血压升高、血糖升高、血脂异常、超重和肥胖。

6. 慢性病预防控制工作：本次调查中指针对调查中涉及的慢性病及其危险因素开展的一系列工作，包括政策倡导和发展、调查与监测、干预与管理、信息分析利用、评估、科学研究。

7. 疾控系统慢性病防控能力：有效、高效、可持续地履行慢性病预防控制领域中适当任务的能力，本次调查包括政策能力、基础配置能力、参与能力、教育培训与指导能力、合作能力、监测与评估、干预能力、科学研究等的综合能力。

8. 基层医疗卫生机构慢性病防控能力：有效、高效、可持续地履行慢性病预防控制领域中适当任务的能力，本部分调查中包括基础配置；培训、指导；项目参与；知识普及；患者、高危人群早期发现；患者、高危人群管理；患者康复等八部分。

9. 慢性病防控政策能力：主要包括政策认定能力、政策制定能力、政策执行能力、政策评估能力和政策调整能力等。考虑到数据的可获得性等因素，本报告只针对各地、各级慢性病防控政策认定能力和制定能力进行分析。

10. 政策认定能力：即将社会问题转化为政策问题的能力。本调查中主要包括，财政经费支持情况、政府领导参与情况和政策倡导情况等三个方面。

11. 政策制定能力：主要以所在地区本级政府或卫生行政部门制定并发布了现行慢性病防控相关规划的情况为衡量。

12. 慢性病防控相关规划：指各级政府或卫生计生等行政部门为防控慢性病及其危险因素而制定的一段时期的政策性文件，包括慢性病防控综合规划、慢性病防控专病规划和针对慢性病危险因素控制的规划。

13. 慢性病防控综合规划：指针对至少 4 类慢性病（心脑血管疾病、恶性肿瘤、糖尿病和慢性病呼吸系统疾病）中的 2 类，含或不含危险因素（烟草使用、不合理膳食、身体活动不足、酒精使用、超重和肥胖、血压升高、血糖升高、血脂异常）均可。

14. 慢性病防控专病规划：指专门针对心脑血管疾病、恶性肿瘤、糖尿病和慢性呼吸系统疾病等慢性病中的一类疾病（含或不含危险因素）制定的规划。针对慢性病危险因素控制的规划指专门针对烟草使用、膳食、身体活动、酒精使用、超重或肥胖、血压、血糖、血脂等危险因素中的任何一项或多项的规划。

15. 慢性病防控基础配置能力：主要包括慢性病防控相关部门、人员、经费、设备等的配置情况。

16. 承担慢性病防控工作的部门：包括三类专门承担慢性病防控工作的部门、以慢性病防控为主要职责的部门和不以慢性病防控为主要职责的部门。

17. 人力资源能力：包括慢性病防控在岗人员数量、年龄分布、工作年限、学历、所学专业和职称等情况。

18. 慢性病防控在岗人员：指 2011 年在岗并承担慢性病防控工作的人员。包括专职人员、承担慢性病防控工作任务的非专职人员，编内和编外人员均计入统计。

19. 基层医疗卫生机构卫生技术在岗人员：包括执业医师、注册护士、药师（士）、检验技师（士）、影像技师（士）、卫生监督员和见习医（药、护、技）师（士）等卫生专业人员，不包括从事管理工作的卫生技术人员（如院长、副院长、党委书记等）。

20. 经费配置能力：主要指被调查疾控中心 2011 年到账的慢性病防控工作经费情况。被调查基层医疗卫生机构 2011 年到账的基本公共卫生服务经费情况。

21. 设备配置能力：主要指基层医疗卫生机构配置慢性病防控相关设备的情况。

22. 慢性病防控教育培训与指导能力：是一个广义的概念，它包括培训能力、指导能力和知识普及能力等 3 个方面。培训能力包括开展培训和参与培训。开展培训，即对慢性病防控工作人员开展相关培训的情况；参与培训，即组织本单位人员参与慢性病防控相关培训的情况。指导能力，即对下级机构开展慢性病防控工作现场指导的情况。知识普及能力指基层医疗卫生机构向大众宣传慢性病防控相关知识的情况。

23. 慢性病防控现场工作（技术）指导：主要指各级疾控中心和基层医疗卫生机构对其技术指导单位开展慢性病防控相关工作（技术）指导的情况。具体包括，省级和地市级疾控中心对县（区）级疾控中心的指导；县（区）级疾控中心对基层医疗卫生机构的指导和基层医疗卫生机构对社区卫生服务站或村卫生室的指导。

24. 知识普及能力：主要指被调查基层医疗卫生机构在慢性病防控相关健康主题日（主要包括世界高血压日、世界糖尿病日、全民健康生活方式日、世界无烟日、世界脑卒中日和世界心脏病日等）期间开展相关知识宣传活动的情况。

25. 慢性病防控合作与参与能力：是一个广义的概念，它包括与其他机构或部门在慢性病防控领域开展项目合作的能力和参与上级机构慢性病防控相关工作的能力。

26. 慢性病监测：主要包括死因监测、慢性病危险因素监测、慢性病发病和患病登记等。慢性病监测能力主要指各级、各地慢性病监测工作的开展情况。

27. 慢性病干预：主要指采取各种措施，控制慢性病和相关危险因素流行，促进慢性病的早期发现和规范管理或延缓慢性病及并发症的发生和发展。慢性病干预与管理主要包括三个环节，危险因素控制、早诊早治和规范化管理。

28. 慢性病干预与管理能力：主要指各级各地危险因素控制、慢性病患者和高危人群早发现及管理工作的开展情况。

29. 慢性病评估能力：主要指对慢性病流行情况及慢性病防控相关工作开展情况的评估能力。

30. 慢性病科研能力：主要指在慢性病防控领域开展科研工作的情况。

31. 高血压患者管理率：2011 年管理高血压患者的人数/高血压患者人数×100%。

高血压患者人数估算：辖区常住人口数×20%（高血压患病率、估算）。

高血压患病率(20%)= 全国高血压患者估算人数(2.66亿)/全国人口数(13.39亿)×100%。

(13.39 亿全国人口数来自第六次人口普查数)；2.66 亿高血压患者数字来自《中国心血管病报告 2012》。

32. 高血压患者规范管理率：2011 年随访四次以上的患者人数/2011 年管理高血压患者人数×100%。

33. 高血压患者控制率：2011 年随访四次以上的患者中最近一次血压达标的人数/2011 年管理高血压患者人数×100%。

34. 糖尿病患者管理率：2011 年管理糖尿病患者的人数/糖尿病患者人数×100%。

糖尿病患者人数估算：辖区常住人口数×18岁以上人群比例×9.7%(糖尿病患病率)。

[糖尿病患病率(9.7%)来源于中国慢性病及其危险因素监测报告(2010)]

35. 糖尿病患者规范管理率：2011 年随访四次以上的患者人数/2011 年管理糖尿病患者

的人数×100%。

36. 糖尿病患者控制率：2011 年随访四次以上的患者中最近一次血糖达标的人数/2011 年管理糖尿病患者的人数×100%。

参 考 文 献

1. 杨功焕 .2008 年全国疾控系统慢性病预防控制能力调查报告. 北京：人民卫生出版社，2010.
2. 梁晓峰，施小明. 中国慢性病预防控制能力调查报告 2009. 北京：人民卫生出版社，2013.
3. 中国疾病预防控制中心，中国疾病预防控制中心慢性非传染性疾病预防控制中心. 中国慢性病及其危险因素监测报告 2010. 北京：军事医学科学出版社，2012.
4. 中华人民共和国卫生部. 中国卫生统计年鉴 2012. 北京：中国协和医科大学出版社，2012.
5. 卫生部. 疾病预防控制工作绩效评估标准（2012 年版）. 2013.
6. 卫生部疾病预防控制局. 全国慢性病预防控制工作规范（试行）2011.
7. 卫生部，等. 中国慢性病防治工作规划（2012~2015 年）. 2012.
8. 卫生部心血管病防治研究中心. 中国心血管病报告 2012. 北京：中国大百科全书出版社，2013.
9. 国家基本公共卫生服务规范（2011 年版）.
10. 司向，翟屹，施小明. 中国慢性非传染性疾病预防控制能力评估. 中华流行病学杂志，2014，35（6）：675-679.
11. 尹香君，施小明，司向，等. 中国疾病预防控制系统慢性非传染性疾病预防控制能力评估. 中华流行病学杂志，2010，31（10）：1125-1129.